T0095724

YOUR GUIDE TO
HOLISTIC BEAUTY

Using the Wisdom of
Traditional Chinese Medicine
Radiant Face, Skin, Hair, Eyes and Health
from the Inside Out

By Zhang Yifang

Better Link Press

This book is edited and designed by the Editorial Committee of *Cultural China* series

Text: Zhang Yifang
Translation: Maurita Dayes
Illustration: Maurita Dayes, Roger Yan, Zhang Yifang
Photos: Zhang Yifang, Liu Shenghui, Quanjing, Ding Guoxing
Cover Design: Wang Wei
Interior Design: Li Jing, Hu Bin (Yuan Yinchang Design Studio)

Copy Editor: Kirstin Mattson, Anna Nguyen
Editor: Yang Xiaohe
Editorial Director: Zhang Yicong

Senior Consultants: Sun Yong, Wu Ying, Yang Xinci
Managing Director and Publisher: Wang Youbu

ISBN: 978-1-60220-152-1

Address any comments about *Your Guide to Holistic Beauty: Using the Wisdom of Traditional Chinese Medicine* to:

Better Link Press
99 Park Ave
New York, NY 10016
USA

or

Shanghai Press and Publishing Development Company
F 7 Donghu Road, Shanghai, China (200031)
Email: comments_betterlinkpress@hotmail.com

Printed in China by Shenzhen Donnelley Printing Co., Ltd.
1 3 5 7 9 10 8 6 4 2

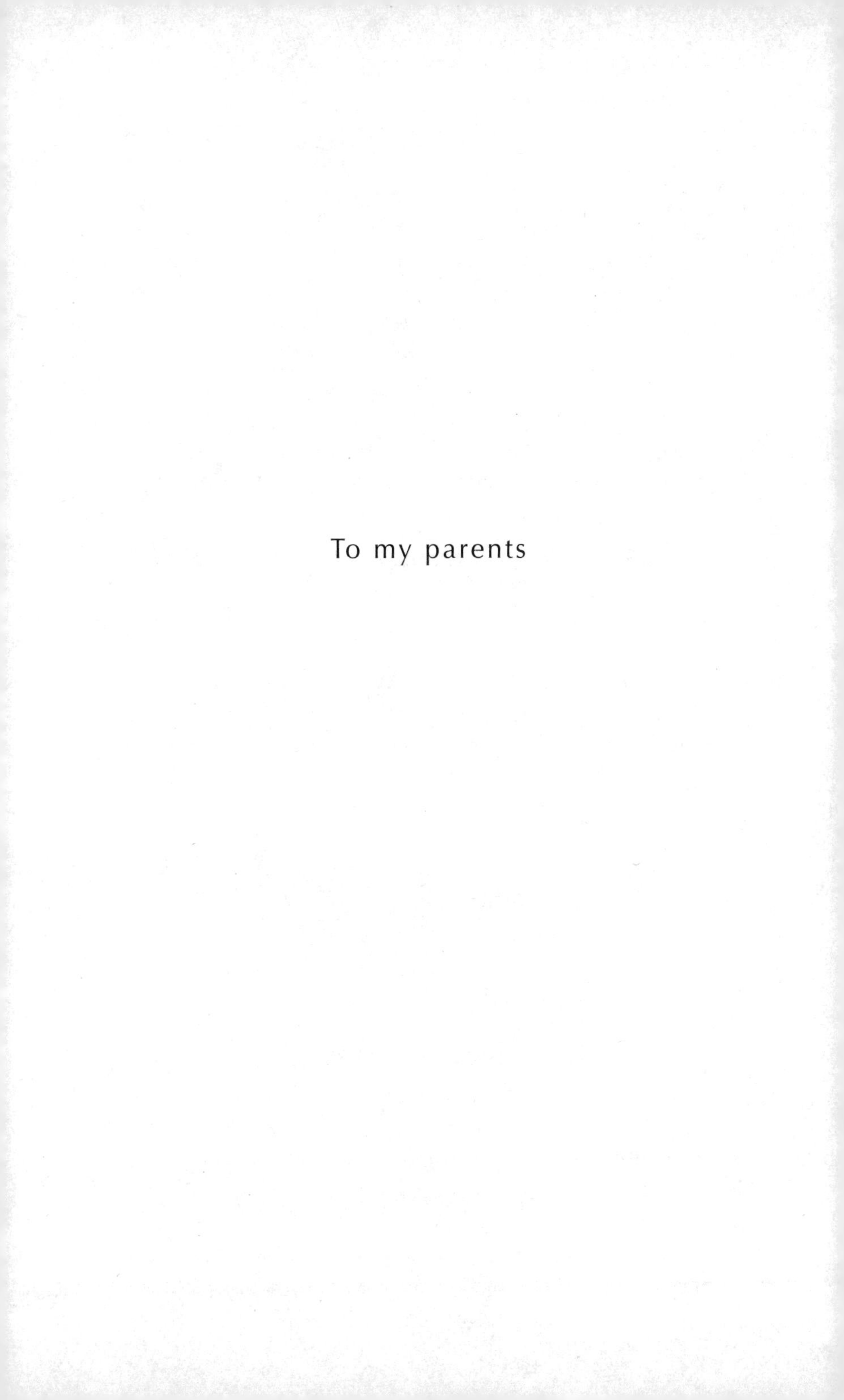

To my parents

Contents

PREFACE 13

ACKNOWLEDGEMENTS 17

INTRODUCTION 19

1. Chinese Perspective on Beauty 19
2. Outer Beauty from Inner Health 21
3. Determining Inner Health from Appearance 22
4. Healthy Skin from a TCM Perspective 23
5. Body Systems as a Tree 24
6. TCM's Natural Approach to Beauty 25

PART ONE
THE CONCEPTS

CHAPTER ONE **Basic TCM Theory and Concepts** 30

1. Chinese View of Organs as a Whole System 30
2. Paired *Zang-Fu* Organs 31
3. The Meridians Connecting the Five Organ Systems 33
4. Organ System Linkages 37
5. Integrated Organ Systems 40
6. Qi, Blood, Body Fluid and the Organ Systems 42
7. External Factors Influencing the Organ Systems 43

CHAPTER TWO **Beauty from the Inside Out** 46

1. Skin 47
2. Hair 55

3. Eyes 60
4. Body Shape 65

CHAPTER THREE Natural Ways to Enhance Beauty 72
1. Food and Herbs 72
2. Self-Massage 74
3. Natural Masks 74
4. Other Options 76
5. Top Ten Super Herbs for Beauty 76

CHAPTER FOUR Self-Assessing Your Five Organ Systems and Body Constitution 97
1. Assessing Your Five Organ Systems 97
2. Assessing Your Body Consitution 101

PART TWO
ORGAN SYSTEM ANALYSIS

CHAPTER FIVE The Heart System 109
1. Basic Facts about the Heart System 110
2. Function of the Physical Heart: Blood and Blood Circulation 110
3. Function of the Mental Heart: Mental Activities and Emotional State 112
4. Meridians of the Heart System 114
5. Heart System and Beauty 116
Face: Flower of the Heart 116
Pulse: Measure of the Heart 117
Tongue: Sprout of the Heart 117
Happiness: Emotion of the Heart 119
6. Beauty Problems and Enhancement 119
Achieving Beautiful Rosy Cheeks 120

1) Imbalance: Redness (with or without Spider Veins) 120
2) Imbalance: Purple Spider Veins (with Facial Redness or Paleness) 123
3) Imbalance: Pale Face 126
Smooth Circulation 127
1) Imbalance: Cold Limbs 127
2) Imbalance: Lymph Edema 129
Healthy Tongue 130
1) Imbalance: Speech Disorder 130
2) Imbalance: Ulcers 131
Sound Sleep 132
1) Imbalance: Insomnia 133
2) Imbalance: Dream Disturbed Sleep 133
3) Imbalance: Sweaty Palms 134

CHAPTER SIX The Liver System 137
1. Basic Facts about the Liver System 138
2. Functions of the Liver 138
Regulate Qi for the Whole Body 138
Storing and Directing Blood 143
3. Meridians of the Liver System 145
4. Liver System and Beauty 146
Eyes and Tears: Window and Liquid of the Liver 146
Breasts: Outer Territory of the Liver 148
Tendons: Tissue of the Liver 149
Nails: Flower of the Liver 150
Skin Color Changes: Signal of Liver Toxin 151
Anger: Emotion of the Liver 152
5. Beauty Problems and Enhancement 153
Enticing Eyes 154
1) Imbalance: Red Eyes 154
2) Imbalance: Itchy Eyes 157
3) Imbalance: Yellow Eyes 158

4) Imbalance: Dry Eyes 159
Beautiful Breasts 161
1) Imbalance: Slow Development or Sagging Breasts 161
2) Imbalance: Early Stage Breast Cysts 164
3) Imbalance: Mastitis 166
4) Imbalance: Breast Lumps (Solid Nodules) 167
Flexible Tendons and Strong Nails 168
1) Imbalance: Weakness of Tendons Breakage and Slow Nail Growth 169
2) Imbalance: Sprained Tendons 170
3) Imbalance: Nail Fungus and Athlete's Foot 170
Healthy Color on the Skin 170
1) Imbalance: Pigmentation after Giving Birth 171
2) Imbalance: White Spots and Vitiligo 172
3) Imbalance: Dark Pigmentation, Purple Dots on the Tongue Company with Dull Ache in the Rib Area 173
Don't Let Anger Build up 174

CHAPTER SEVEN The Spleen System 177
1. Basic Facts about the Spleen System 178
2. Functions of the Spleen 178
"Transformation": Separating Nutrition and Waste 179
"Transportation": Ascending the "Clear" 179
"Transportation": Descending the Waste 180
Governing the Blood Flow within the Vessels 181
3. Meridians of the Spleen System 183
4. Spleen System and Beauty 184
Mouth: the "Opening" of the Spleen 185
Saliva: Helping Digestion 187
Lips: Flower of the Spleen 188
Muscles: Tissue of the Spleen 189
Limbs: Outer Territory of the Spleen 190
Thinking and Longing: Emotion of

the Spleen 190
5. Beauty Problems and Enhancement 192
Staying Fit 192
1) Imbalance: Water Retention and Edema 192
2) Imbalance: Cellulite 197
3) Imbalance: Overweight 198
4) Imbalance: Underweight 199
5) Imbalance: Saggy Skin 200
Terrific Tummy 202
1) Imbalance: Constipation 203
2) Imbalance: Bloating 204
3) Imbalance: Diarrhea 205
Fresh Breath and Luscious Lips 206
1) Imbalance: Bad Breath 206
2) Imbalance: Pale or Purple Lips 207
3) Imbalance: Cracked Lips or Canker Sores 208
4) Imbalance: Under Eye Bags 209

CHAPTER EIGHT The Lung System 211
1. Basic Facts about the Lung System 212
2. Functions of the Lung 212
Body's First Line of Defense 212
Governing Respiration 213
Regulating Body Fluid 214
Facilitating Convergence of the Blood Vessels 215
Governing Qi 216
3. Meridians of the Lung System 219
4. Lung System and Beauty 221
Skin and Body Hair: Reflection of Lung Function 222
Nose: "Opening" of the Lung 224
Larynx: Passageway for Oxygen to Enter the Lung 225
Worry and Sadness: Emotions of the Lung 226
5. Beauty Problems and Enhancement 228

Sensational Skin 228
1) Imbalance: Dry Skin 228
2) Imbalance: Sensitive Skin 232
3) Imbalance: Rashes and Lumps 232
4) Imbalance: Acne 234
5) Imbalance: Warts 235
6) Imbalance: Pigmentation 236
Healthy Nose 237
1) Imbalance: Sinus 237
2) Imbalance: Running Nose 238
3) Imbalance: Nosebleeds 238
4) Imbalance: Rosacea, Redness and Swelling of the Nose 239
Fluid Metabolism 239
1) Imbalance: Puffy Face 239
2) Imbalance: Hoarse Voice 241

CHAPTER NINE The Kidney System 243
1. Basic Facts about the Kidney System 244
2. Functions of the Kidney 244
Storing and Releasing Congenital and Acquired Essence 245
1) Types of Essence and the Basic Functions 245
2) Facilitating the Body's Development and Growth 246
3) Creating Yin-Yang Balance 251
Governing Water Metabolism 252
1) Reusing Body Fluid and Dispelling Waste 252
2) Promoting Water Metabolism for Other Organs 254
3) Governing the Reception of Qi 254
3. Meridians of the Kidney System 256
4. Kidney System and Beauty 258
Bones: Tissue of the Kidney 258
Ears: Window of the Kidney 260
Lower Orifices: A Link to the Kidney 261

Thick Saliva: Controlled by the Kidney 261
Hair: Flower of Kidney 262
Fear and Fright: Emotions of the Kidney 263
5. Beauty Problems and Enhancement 265
Heavenly Hair 265
Anti-Aging 271
1) Imbalance: Weaker Teeth 271
2) Imbalance: Hearing Loss or Tinnitus 272
3) Imbalance: Joint Weaknesses and Posture 273
4) Imbalance: Lower Back Pain 274
Sex life 275
1) Imbalance: Pelvic Floor Dysfunction 275
2) Imbalance: Low Sexual Drive 276
3) Imbalance: Hemorrhoids 276
4) Imbalance: Erectile Dysfunction 277

APPENDICES 279
Getting Ready: Preparing Your Kitchen Tools and Ingredients 279
Cooking Techniques 280
Meridian Database: Illustrations, Acupuncture Points and Locations 282
TCM Glossary 301
Bibliography 307
Index 309
A Useful Guide to Foods and Herbs: Considering Constitution and Organ System *Gatefold*

PREFACE

Finding a way to maintain a positive spirit, healthy lifestyle and youthful look has become an important focus these days, and people are increasingly looking to natural methods to attain these goals. Traditional Chinese medicine (TCM) provides a time-honored way to achieve and maintain health, and holds that through inner health we can improve outward appearance as well. The keys to beauty lie within.

Our face, eyes, skin and hair all contribute to appearance, and TCM shows us how to keep them looking their best. It is undeniable that being good looking and radiating health is a common goal. Research shows that attractive people get better jobs and more pay, and have an advantage in relationships. However the importance of outward appearance goes much deeper. It shows what is going on inside the body, and allows us to address health problems before they become critical, enhancing quality of life and increasing longevity.

Around the globe, over countless years, people have pursued youthful vitality and beauty utilizing a multitude of methods. Nowadays this often takes the form of supplements in pill, powder or liquid form, or topical treatments. TCM moves beyond the superficial, believing in the importance of the overall function of the organ systems influenced by qi (the body's vital energy), blood and body fluid, and harmony between the mind, body and surrounding environment. It employs natural solutions, including food and herb remedies and massage, and emphasizes the importance of a healthy lifestyle, including sunlight, relaxation and sound sleep.

This book will give you essential information about holistic beauty, teaching simple and effective TCM practices that will put you on the path to resolve the beauty issues in your daily life.

I have written this book for three reasons. To begin with, I realized that we are continually faced with decisions regarding long-term beauty, and we need information in order to make the right choices. These include whether to go to a salon, apply skin care products and cosmetics, undergo plastic surgery or undertake holistic care. Holistic care is the most comprehensive and natural, focusing on three aspects: having a good appetite and individualized diet plan, sleeping soundly and regularly, and maintaining normal elimination (such as sweat, urine, stool, ejaculation and menstruation).

If acne or pimples on appear on the face, or a rash on the skin, this is the body trying to communicate with you. It is signaling you, warning: "Aha, you need to take care of your lifestyle!" The outward manifestations might result from stress and burn-out, not having enough sleep, improper diet, irritable bowel syndrome or disharmony of the reproductive system.

You must find the root cause and resolve it, not merely treat its symptom. If you can't find the cause by yourself, you can seek a professional's help, but to solve the inner problem, not to hide or cover it. This sign shouldn't be ignored; if we can see what is coming and nip it in the bud, this will help not only with beauty issues but overall health.

One of my patients had a cyst, about the size of a ping pong ball, on his right knee. After examination by CT scan, his surgeon had suggested an operation. He came to me for a second opinion, and after consultation, I diagnosed that his blood circulation needed some adjustment. He received a series of acupuncture treatments, and combined with some healthy changes to his diet and lifestyle, the cyst completely disappeared within three months without surgery.

Another example was a patient who did not have the habit of drinking water and eating proper breakfasts. He was anxious when he came to see me, as a lump had developed behind his left ear. I found that he had improper fluid metabolism as well as stagnation of phlegm. By simply increasing his warm water intake in the morning and adding some foods to remove phlegm blockage, his lump disappeared after a few weeks.

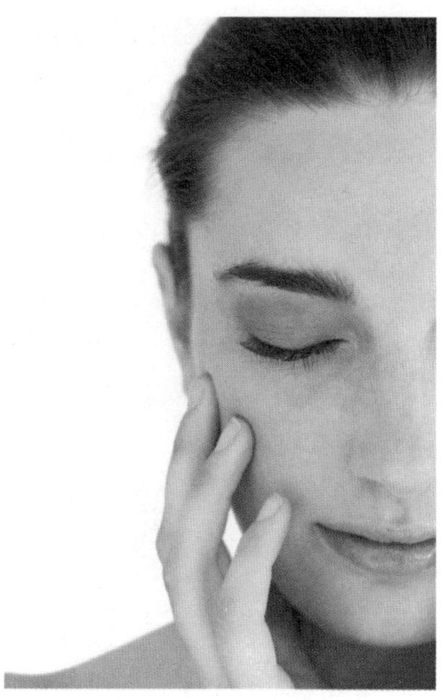

Fig. 1 Find and treat the root cause of beauty problems and achieve holistic beauty.

The second reason for writing this book comes from wanting to share my family's history of many simple yet effective remedies to treat beauty-related issues. Speaking personally, I could not tolerate spicy foods and wine, and I would easily get red in the face and rashes on my skin if I ingested a small amount. Instead of ignoring it, I used a TCM method to prevent it and harmonize my body. I drink cold smoked plum tea in summer, or warm hawthorn berry tea in winter, before I attend public events or social activities. By doing so I can enjoy myself without worrying about suffering from those physical conditions.

As another example, when I turned 42 years old, I started to see grey hair. It showed a lot since my hair is dark black. I talked to my mother, and she said she did not have any grey hair until after 50. This made me think about underlying causes; in particular, was there anything I did that weakened my kidney? I started to experience a lot of back and joint pain in addition to this beauty issue. I consulted my father, a TCM practitioner, who said I had spleen and kidney disharmony. I knew I had to take action. I decided to follow natural rhythms and sleep around 11 p.m., rather than drinking tea to hold off sleepiness and continuing to study and work, as I had in the past. In addition, I undertook a regime of massaging my head two to three times a week, and eating black sesame seeds and walnut powder in winter for two months. Fifteen years later, I still do not have much grey hair.

Last but not least, I wanted to draw attention to the many diagnostic skills and treatments that can enhance beauty through both inner harmony and outer care. These important ways to allow people to obtain health, happiness and beauty using TCM have not yet drawn the wide attention of the global medical field.

This book uses case studies, system assessments, treatment details, recipes and illustrations to help you manage your health and beauty issues. Combined with my previous two books, this will give you the information you need to understand yourself, build an individualized treatment program, and move toward long-term radiant health and a joyful life.

The material in this book is provided for informational purposes only and is not intended as medical advice. This book should not be used as a sole source of information to diagnose or treat any illness, disorder, disease, or health problem. Always consult your physician or health care provider before beginning treatment for a medical condition.

I am so happy to have the chance to make these introductory remarks to set you on your way, and am eager to share ancient traditions that have not been available previously in English. The theory and techniques of TCM are a gift to the whole world. I hope you will come on the journey with me, and discover new tools to enhance your beauty and enjoy lasting health with your family and friends.

Dr. Zhang Yifang

ACKNOWLEDGEMENTS

Combining my personal experiences from last 30 years with the knowledge and practices of TCM that have developed during its 5000-year history, this book is a fruit of my studies and accumulation on Chinese medical holistic beauty.

My highest gratitude goes to my mother Jiang Danru and father Zhang Jize, who always encourage me to share my knowledge globally. Many of the skin and hair care tips I have learned from my mother, and the foods, herb remedies, and recipes were taught to me by my father. My parents will celebrate their diamond marriage this year. Hereinafter, I would like to present this book as my gift to them. I wish them happiness, health, and longevity!

I want to especially thank Maurita Dayes for helping me translate the context of this book into written English and also her contribution to many of the original ideas, including the analogy of the trees, up-to-date research information, and the utilization of essential oils. I would really like to extend my appreciation to all the lovely hand-drawn watercolor paintings, which have taken a lot of her time and efforts, and helped to bring my words to life. They created an atmosphere where art and medicine can coexist.

Thanks to Professor and Chief Doctor Zhang Ming from Yueyang Hospital Shanghai who contributed her knowledge of facial Chinese medical therapy and herbs for acne and pigmentation. Professor Yao Yingzhi from Nanjing University of Chinese Medicine who shared her knowledge with me about beauty herbs and pictures. My thanks also goes to Roger Yan, a friend and an innovative artist, who created the meridian and massage drawings for this book.

Special thanks to my husband Wu Jianwei for his valuable suggestions, great encouragement, and editing assistance. Many thanks to my daughter Wu Mengyue. She recommended some TCM beauty books for me, and spent days finding references and information.

Great thanks goes to our editor Yang Xiaohe for her patience and support, guidance, and effective communication. Thanks to Kirstin Mattson for her editorial talents and logical approach, and she bears my precious memory for editing my three books. On the whole, this book would have been impossible to write without everybody's contributions.

According to the Chinese saying, *xiao yi xiao, shi nian shao,* smiling has magic results for our body and mood. A young appearance has a positive impact on our mental and physical health. Let us smile when we wake up every morning, keep a young heart, and then receive a reward of looking beautiful or handsome each day.

In order to use this book more efficiently and effectively, readers may also get some additional information from my website, www.acherbs.com, and my previous two books, *Using Traditional Chinese Medicine to Manage Your Emotional Health* and *Your Guide to Health with Foods & Herbs*.

Wishing health, happiness, and a radiant appearance for you, your family, and your friends.

Dr. Zhang Yifang

INTRODUCTION

Well-being, longevity and beauty have all been enhanced, for countless generations, by those astute enough to use the ancient but effective practice of traditional Chinese medicine (TCM).

In this book, we will explore how to create health, and therefore beauty, from the inside out, so that your face, hair, eyes, skin, nails and every element of your being are functioning optimally. As you implement some of the concepts in this book, you will find that focusing on inner health using strategies from TCM can produce outstanding results in your appearance.

This book is not just for women. Many beauty books are written with only women in mind, since traditionally the beauty industry has been geared toward women. However, since superior health and looking your best are relevant topics for men as well, this book is for men and women alike.

Yes, you will learn how to look fabulous! However this book does not address beauty concerns at a superficial level, instead exploring how to develop radiant health throughout every cell in your body. As the traditional saying goes, *yi nei yang wai*—nourish the inside so it shines outwardly.

1. Chinese Perspective on Beauty

Beauty is difficult to define, since beauty is truly "in the eye of the beholder" and is interpreted differently across various cultures. While it is tempting to limit the definition to what the surrounding culture deems as beautiful, assigning one particular ideal is simply too limiting.

The fact is, our concept of beauty changes due to factors such as time, economic status and fads that come and go. In Western culture alone, history has shown that during many times of economic instability, when the majority of the population was concerned with meeting basic needs, a voluptuous figure for women was more desirable than a skinny one. Curves were envied since most people did not have the means to achieve this full figured look. During the 1970s and 80s, the skinny, waif look became popular throughout most Western cultures, only to be replaced in the 90s when the voluptuous figure made a comeback once again. So the cycle continues.

The idea that the perception of what is beautiful changes with time has been long understood in Chinese culture. *Huan fei Yan shou* is a common saying in China, meaning "different time, different beauty". Huan and Yan are the names of two famous women from different dynasties who were legends because of their exceptional beauty. *Fei* means fleshy and *shou* means skinny. Huan refers to Yang Yuhuan (719–756), who lived during the Tang dynasty. Described as voluptuous, she was a role model for women everywhere at that time, and everybody wanted to be like her. On the other hand, Zhao Feiyan (45 BC–1 BC), who lived during the Han dynasty and was famous for her dancing, was known to be skinny with a no muscle, no fat look. Women of that time desired to emulate her appearance. So this popular saying means that ideal beauty can change, influenced by a variety of cultural factors at a specific point in time.

Then how can we truly define it? What elements of beauty remain consistent in every culture and every period of time? Some universal factors, evident in a body seen to be flourishing, include:

- Shiny, thick, fast-growing hair
- Clear, bright eyes
- Radiant, hydrated and blemish-free skin on the face and body
- A balanced and coordinated physique
- Clear sinus passages

- White, shiny teeth
- Firm, elastic muscles
- Rosy, nourished and smooth lips
- Well-rounded, shiny and strong nails
- Even eyebrows

These are some of the markers that indicate a certain harmony. And of course there are markers of disharmony, commonly thought of as displeasing to the eye, such as edema, hair loss or pimples, to name a few.

2. Outer Beauty from Inner Health

What remains eternally beautiful is health. Health from deep within the body generates an outer glow that is translated into something we cannot define with words. It is that feeling you have when you see someone and think, "Wow, what a stunning person." This person may or may not have "classic" beauty or possess the golden triangle, that illusive mathematical equation of perfect dimensions. But the person is stunning because something shines through everywhere—a combination of a healthy body within and a beautiful spirit that comes from a balanced mind.

This leads to the well-established maxim that true beauty is more than skin deep. Practicing TCM leads us to knowledge about the connections of the inside to the outside, and new discoveries about our bodies. For instance, it is largely unknown that addressing spleen dysfunction, deep within the body, can help to correct edema, cellulite and sagging skin.

In this book you will discover how traditional Chinese medicine identifies your five organ systems, which are quite different than the organs as viewed by Western medicine. Keeping these systems healthy is vital, as they have a profound impact on outer beauty. The starring role they play is the foundation for this book. The five organ systems, and how they play an integral role in the maintenance of a healthy body and mind, will be examined in-depth.

In addition, beauty rituals that have long been used in China will be examined. These protocols have been thoroughly tried and tested over thousands of years. They are ethical (they required no animal testing as men and women used them on themselves) and effective strategies, which have been documented and passed on to the following generations, as others deemed ineffective were refined or laid aside. Each and every dynasty added to the beauty and wellness regiments of the previous ones. The treatments included things that could be eaten, applied to their skin, and so much more.

These methods are safe, natural and have been proven to be successful over a period of 5000 years. There are detox protocols, prescriptions for healing, and many other treasures that have played a role in enhancing health, longevity and beauty throughout China's long history. After reading this book you will have a thorough understanding of how to regulate your body using holistic concepts and make accurate assessments based on syndrome identification.

3. Determining Inner Health from Appearance

Your outward appearance can speak volumes about your inner health. Our most frustrating beauty concerns often are urgent messages from our body, communicating the need for some care and attention.

In the West, the appearance of a wrinkle is often seen as an inevitable sign that the ravages of time have taken their toll. But according to TCM, spots or wrinkles that appear in certain places may be providing information about the health of a particular organ. When that organ is rebalanced, some of these lines will disappear. Even hair loss is a popular topic addressed in Chinese medical chronicles, treating it through correcting internal imbalances.

When a TCM doctor does a consultation, what the patient verbally communicates about symptoms is not the only source of information. The doctor is also taking note of other markers of health, such as the skin, hair, eyes, tongue, nose, mouth and lips. Furthermore the patient's mannerisms will be taken into consideration when diagnosing internal well-being or underlying dysfunction. A simple example is the presence of rosy cheeks and lips, which may indicate good circulation of qi (the body's vital energy) and blood making its way to the head. The nails and tongue are another indication of health, and will often be observed.

Consider the elasticity of the skin and muscles. In TCM, the spleen influences muscle integrity, so muscular issues can indicate spleen dysfunction. Similarly the skin is dependent upon a healthy lung system and circulation. Healthy skin, hair and nails have a particular quality to them; they shine and have a certain depth, like fine jade. They speak about the health of your internal organs.

4. Healthy Skin from a TCM Perspective

Let's begin by discussing the skin since it covers the largest surface of the body.

Traditionally, TCM practitioners would observe the color, hydration and radiance of the skin. In addition, doctors now look at skin elasticity, which also communicates subtle messages about internal functions. So what should healthy skin look like from a TCM perspective?

Firstly, the underlying color is important. A rosy tint beneath the surface might indicate good blood circulation, but a new or unusual yellow tinge to the skin (besides that which is congenital) can often communicate issues with the liver or spleen.

Secondly, healthy skin has the ability to maintain hydration. Why is it that after staying in the sun for just half an hour, some people develop dry, red and irritated skin? Of course certain skin types can better tolerate the sun than others, but that is not what is meant here. The important factor is the skin's ability to retain adequate water to protect it from the sun's dehydrating effects. Having skin with optimal levels of fatty protein will help hold moisture and can stop it from drying out. The fatty protein levels in the skin are dependent upon diet, but also relate to the organ systems and their ability to transform and transport this nourishment to every part of the body.

A radiant complexion is another important factor for enviable skin. According to Chinese medicine, a complexion that glows is a result of a harmonized body and soul. It is the product of a healthy spirit, combined with the essence with which you were born and the essence you have accumulated throughout your lifetime. Essence, as defined by TCM, is created when blood circulation, qi/energy and body fluid are flowing optimally, bringing nourishment to every part of the body. Therefore good circulation and the movement of qi, blood and body fluids (including lymph) are important factors.

5. Body Systems as a Tree

Have you ever taken the time to just lie beneath a giant tree and appreciate its beauty? You might notice the sunshine bounce from leaf to leaf as the branches sway gently in the wind. It might surprise you that nearly every leaf is a different shade of green and some are not even green at all. Upon closer inspection of a delicate leaf, you might observe the intricate network of veins that bring nourishment and hydration all the way from the ground so that each leaf develops a healthy deep, rich color. If you are lucky your tree might be filled with flowers.

In appreciating the beauty of a tree, our focus is usually on the leaves and flowers. We rarely take time to think about the trunk and the roots because they are not as pretty or are out of sight. It is the root system, however, that brings the nourishment to the leaves and branches. This nourishment travels up through the roots, into the trunk, and up a network of pathways to reach every last part of the tree. The root system travels deep into the soil to seek out what is needed to make the tree thrive.

This illustration (fig. 2) helps to explain a traditional way

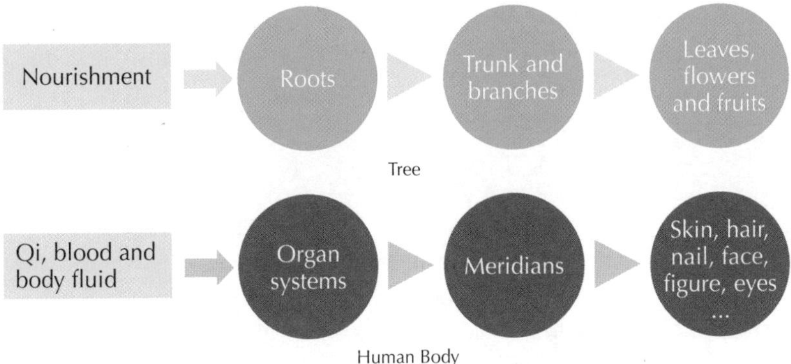

Fig. 2 Tree system and the human body

that TCM approaches beauty. The vitality of the tree is absolutely dependent on a healthy root system and the ability of this system to deliver nutrition to each and every part of the tree. Those parts starved of nourishment die off or become blemished.

It is not so different with our bodies. We are reliant upon the health of our inner organ systems and their ability to deliver nourishment to every extremity.

6. TCM's Natural Approach to Beauty

Modern nutrition addresses imbalances through diet and by supplements of vitamins and minerals in pill, powder or liquid form. Chinese medicine places a greater emphasis on the nourishment and regulation of entire body systems and their interrelationship with the body's inner terrain and outer environment. The use of herbs, food and physical therapies can be used to support the organ systems, ultimately correcting imbalances that have occurred.

While the Western practice of nutrition has focused on researching the function of different vitamins and minerals and their effect on the health of the human body, Chinese medicine focuses on the five organ systems (about which we will learn more shortly). It follows the belief that the overall function of these systems, influenced by qi, blood and body fluid, is far more important.

Food and herbal medicine are only part of the picture. Their therapeutic use becomes more effective when combined with external manipulation of the organ systems through the stimulation of meridians, channels and acupressure/acupuncture points, which are conduits for the flow of vital energy. In addition any therapy has much better results when combined with healthy lifestyle practices such as getting enough sunlight, relaxation and beauty sleep.

Let's take a few minutes to discuss the concepts of qi, blood, body fluids and meridians according to TCM.

Chinese medicine holds that everything is made out of qi. When qi is collected it may form solid materials such internal body structures, flesh, or even trees and other things in nature. When qi is unstructured it is an invisible force with robust power and movement. Blood is well known as the red nutritious fluid that flows in the blood vessels, but it also flows in the meridians. Body fluid is a general term for all the liquid within the body including lymphatic liquid.

Qi, blood and body fluids are the most fundamental substances comprising the human body. Qi contributes to making up your body structures, and flows within your body in an invisible form, along with the visible blood and body fluids. Without these three essential substances you would not be alive.

Meridians and collaterals are the pathways through which qi, blood and body fluids circulate. They also serve as the interconnections between the viscera and the limbs, making it possible for the upper and lower, as well as the internal and external, portions of the body to communicate with each other.

According to TCM, when energy is weak in function or lacking in quantity or quality, or if there is insufficient blood or body fluid inside the organ systems, then dull, saggy skin and muscles may occur. Furthermore, a pale face or the accumulation of pigmentation might be observed. In order to maintain a radiant complexion, and remain youthful and physically active as one

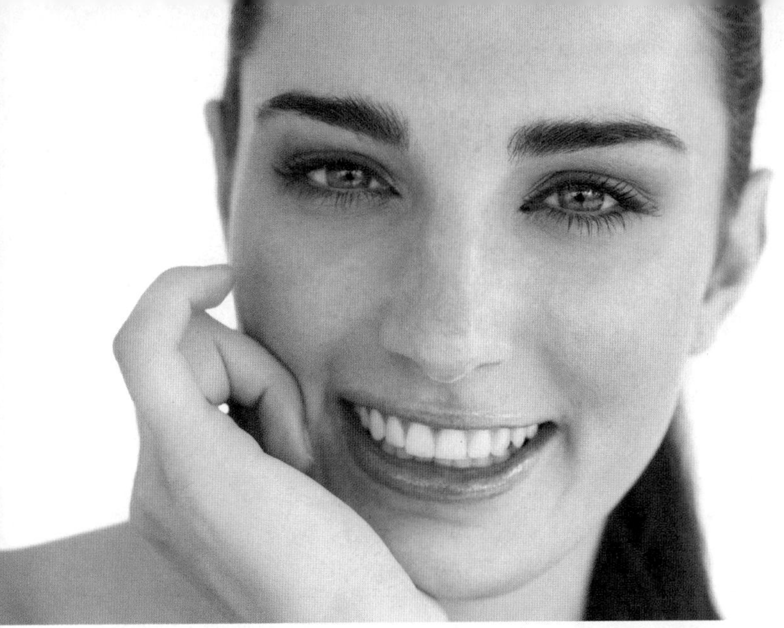

Fig. 3 TCM approaches beauty-related issues through the regulation of the organ systems.

ages, TCM approaches beauty issues through the regulation of the organ systems. These include the use of food, herbal medicine, acupressure, acupuncture, *gua sha* (a technique of scraping the surface of the skin with jade in order to remove stagnation), skin masks, tinctures, pastes, herbal baths and herbal foot baths (fig. 3). These techniques can influence the energy, blood and body fluid within the organs and meridians.

There is a lovely traditional Chinese saying:

Rosy cheeks are the flower of the heart
Beautiful lips are the flower of the spleen
Beautiful nails are the flower of the liver
Shiny, elastic, soft and long hair is the flower of the kidney
Beautiful skin is the flower of the lung
Take care of your roots and your flowers will be beautiful.

We need to spend more time and energy focusing on the unseen parts of the body so that the observable parts are perceived to be flourishing and radiating beauty.

PART ONE

THE CONCEPTS

CHAPTER ONE
Basic TCM Theory and Concepts

This chapter provides a brief introduction to TCM's way of viewing the organs and their interrelationships. This information is necessary to fully understand how the liver, spleen, kidney, lung and heart systems influence our appearance.

1. Chinese View of Organs as a Whole System

We first need to explore some fundamental differences between TCM's view of the form and function of organs and the Western anatomical or medical description. When referring to the liver, for example, in Western medicine this means the anatomical organ itself and its function. In Chinese medicine, when we refer to the liver, this includes the whole organ system:

- Structure and function of the organ
- The paired organ
- Related meridians
- The tissue
- Related sense organs
- Emotions unique to that organ
- Sound associated with the organ
- Exterior appearance related to the organ

Therefore if the liver system became imbalanced, issues

might manifest as a problem in any of the areas mentioned above. A good TCM practitioner will recognize the symptoms and prevent a more serious disease from occurring.

2. Paired *Zang-Fu* Organs

In TCM the organs are organized into two categories: *zang* and *fu*.

Let's talk about the *zang* organs first. There are six *zang* organs: the five main organs comprising the heart, lung, liver, spleen and kidney, along with the pericardium. The word "*zang*" in Chinese means "storage", and this is one of the primary functions of this type of organ. We will focus on the five main *zang* organs—heart, lung, liver, spleen and kidney—in depth in this book.

The common physical function of *zang* organs is to produce and store the body's blood, fluid and qi. These organs are responsible for ensuring the body is full of essence and qi, vital and ready for action, and to ensure the flow is not stagnated or blocked. Stagnation or depletion of the qi or essence in an organ can affect overall health and may lead to more serious disease. Without the constant manufacture, distribution and movement of essence and qi, beauty will also be compromised.

The six *fu* organs are: stomach, gallbladder, small intestine, large intestine, urinary bladder and *san jiao*. *San jiao*, meaning "triple energies" or "triple heater", is not one particular anatomical organ. It relates to all muscles and tissues, like a water pipe to carry body fluid, including lymphatic fluid, circulating it to whole body.

In Chinese a *fu* organ is a receptor organ, responsible for receiving food and allowing it to

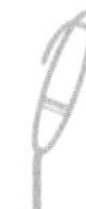

Notes

Although we have a pair of kidneys and lungs, they are referred to singularly as the kidney or lung in TCM.

pass through. So the job of the *fu* organs is to receive solid and liquid food, extract the good and expel the bad.

One vital aspect of the *fu* organs is that there is constant movement. When one organ is full the others need to be empty and in wait. For instance when the stomach is full, the intestines should be empty, waiting for food and vice versa.

Another significant concept about the *fu* organs is that their energy moves downward. For example, since the energy of the stomach needs to be moving downward, if this natural pattern is disturbed and the energy begins moving upward, one might experience indigestion or acid reflux.

It is also important that the *zang* and *fu* organs work together to produce enough nutrition to create and maintain a healthy, harmonized body. When they are working in harmony, the food or liquid that enters the body will be separated into nourishment and waste. The nutrition will be absorbed and distributed into the whole body's systems, while the waste will be excreted.

The *zang* and *fu* organs are also classified into pairs:

Main Paired Organs in TCM

***Zang* Organ**	***Fu* Organ**
Heart	Small intestine
Liver	Gallbladder
Spleen	Stomach
Lung	Large intestine
Kidney	Urinary bladder

The pairing systems of *zang* and *fu* organs developed as a result of three observations.

- Proximity: For instance, the liver is close to the gallbladder, the stomach is close to the spleen, and the kidney is close to the urinary bladder.

- Patterns: These were observed over thousands of years of experience. For instance, it was noted that the lung and large intestine share a special relationship. When one showed patterns of disharmony, the other was often affected, so by treating one you could affect the other.
- Meridians: These pairs are linked by meridians.

3. The Meridians Connecting the Five Organ Systems

Each organ has its own pathway system to carry and transport material to every cell and extremity of the body.

The pathways consist of meridians, or channels, which branch out into collaterals (fig. 4). It is on the superficial meridian where we find the acupuncture points. The deep collaterals have points that cannot be reached with techniques such as acupuncture or other manual modalities. The meridians are where we apply massage, acupressure or acupuncture to rebalance the body. However you can impact the collaterals and the related organ by stimulating acupoints on the meridians. The meridians will also have branches that are less closely linked to other organs.

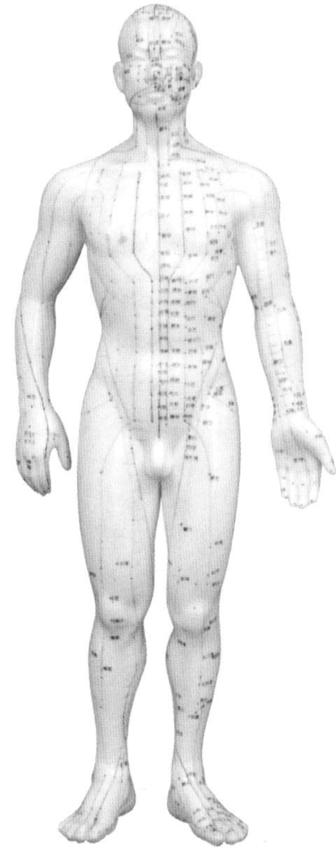

Fig. 4 Meridians and collaterals of the human body

The organs are connected with surface points on the body along these lines of energy. Therefore the entire body, inside and out, comprises one whole system, which moves energy and regulates health.

The saying "you are what you eat" implies a one-sided relationship: the food we eat influences our body composition and health. In other words, something from outside affects the inside. Meridians, however, can go both ways: what we take into our bodies has an effect on outward appearance, while external manipulations on the body surface can influence the functioning of internal organs.

The Meridians

Meridians are energy networks functioning as a transportation system, carrying information to and from each organ. Meridians also transport qi, blood, body fluids, essence and nutrition to every part of the body. There are twelve paired meridians, relating to the *zang* and *fu* organs, as well as two single meridians, relating to the Governing Vessel and Conception Vessel, the main rivers of the body's yin and yang energies.

According to TCM, the external belongs to yang, which together with yin are the balancing forces in nature. In general, yang is associated with the male, the active and heat. The external can be subdivided into the three yang meridian channels: Taiyang, Yangming and Shaoyang. Yang meridians are found on the back of the hands, the outside of the arms and legs, and the back of the trunk. They can influence our *fu* organs.

The internal belongs to yin, traditionally associated with the female, the dark and cold. It can also be further divided into the three yin meridian channels: Taiyin, Shaoyin and Jueyin. Yin meridians are distributed on the palm side of the hands, the inside of the arms and legs, and the front of the trunk. They can influence our *zang* organs.

For instance if there is an exterior manifestation such as pigmentation on the face, we will conduct treatment on yang meridians points on which to conduct treatment, because they travel to the face.

Categories of Meridians		
Category	**Sub-category**	**Meridian**
Yang	Taiyang	Taiyang Bladder Meridian of Foot
		Taiyang Small Intestine Meridian of Hand
	Yangming	Yangming Large Intestine Meridian of Hand
		Yangming Stomach Meridian of Foot
	Shaoyang	Shaoyang Gallbladder Meridian of Foot
		Shaoyang *San Jiao* Meridian of Hand
Yin	Taiyin	Taiyin Lung Meridian of Hand
		Taiyin Spleen Meridian of Foot
	Shaoyin	Shaoyin Heart Meridian of Hand
		Shaoyin Kidney Meridian of Foot
	Jueyin	Jueyin Liver Meridian of Foot
		Jueyin Pericardium Meridian of Hand

One way to understand the relationship between the inside and outside of the body is to think about the effect of a massage. After a massage, most people don't just feel relaxation in their skin or outer muscles, but also have an overall sense of well-being. Manipulating the body's surface energy level is good for the inside of the body as well.

There are many other examples of this linkage, including the practice of holding premature babies to strengthen their immune systems and of energy-healing techniques such as Reiki. Reiki is a type of therapy in which the practitioner uses his or her own energy to change the patient's energy. This occurs without touching the patient, and is similar to Qigong therapy. The intimate touch between lovers, or even just hugging, is another example of how surface contact can provide multiple levels of healing deep within the body.

In order to ensure total health and harmony between the outside and inside, we need to use both external approaches (acupressure and acupuncture) and internal approaches (food and herbs). In this way we can regulate the whole system and achieve overall balance.

The Concept of *San Jiao*

We have previously touched on *san jiao*, one of the *fu* organs, and now will learn more. From head to toe, the body can be divided into three portions, called *san jiao* or triple energies (fig. 5):

- The upper portion of *san jiao* includes the head, arms and chest cavity above the diaphragm, where the heart and lung are located.
- The middle portion corresponds to the region below the diaphragm but above the umbilicus, where the stomach and spleen are located.
- The lower portion is comprised of everything below the umbilicus: functionally this includes the small and large intestines, liver, kidney, bladder and legs.

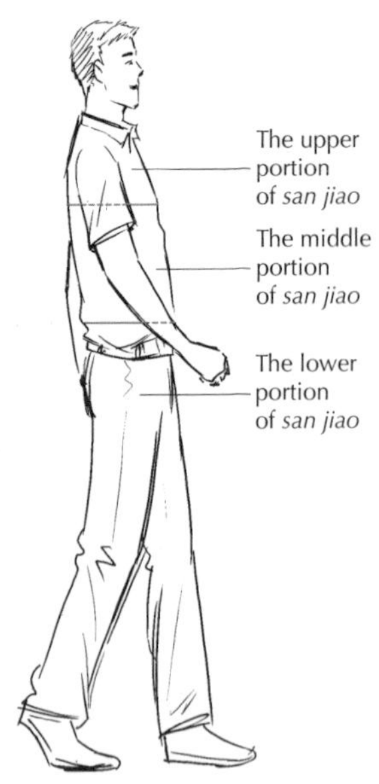

Fig. 5 Location of *san jiao*

Disease typically moves from the upper to the lower portion of *san jiao*. This means it transfers from superficial to deeper levels, and as it does so, it changes from a deficiency to a serious disease.

Since *san jiao* is considered a *fu* organ, it has its own meridian among the twelve standard meridians, and it is paired with the pericardium. Original qi and body fluids circulate within the *san jiao* meridian.

4. Organ System Linkages

A core belief related to TCM is Five Elements Theory, which holds that everything in the universe and within our own bodies can be classified into five groups: wood, fire, earth, metal and water. According to this principle, wood relates to the liver, fire to the heart, earth to the spleen, metal to the lung, and water to the kidney. By using Five Elements Theory and the interrelationship between the organs, we can create balance in our practices to maintain health and beauty.

Organ System Map

	Heart System	Liver System	Spleen System	Lung System	Kidney System
Element	Fire	Wood	Earth	Metal	Water
Emotion	Joy	Anger	Thinking	Sadness	Fear
Sound	Laughing	Shouting	Singing	Crying	Groaning
Tissues	Vessels	Tendons	Muscles	Skin	Bones, teeth
Sense organs	Tongue	Eyes	Mouth	Nose	Ear, lower orifices
External Point of appearance	Face	Nails	Lips	Body hair	Hair
Liquid	Nervous sweat	Tears	Thin saliva	Nasal liquid	Thick saliva

Emotions

It is important to realize that in TCM, the emotions are inextricably linked to the body and cannot be separated. Healthy or negative emotions can affect the organs, while dysfunction in the organs can affect the emotions.

In fact, this emotional element was considered so powerful that in the past, someone struggling with a particular emotion would go to a TCM doctor. Psychology is a relatively new concept in China because TCM acknowledges the intimate relationship between the organs and one's emotions, and it has been effective in treating and harmonizing emotional issues related to organ health. It is still a popular alternative to conventional Western treatments and is used throughout China to this day.

In China we say, "The joys or sorrows of life may eventually show up on the face." Those who are content and determined to enjoy their life habitually have more peaceful expressions on their faces, resulting in a glowing complexion. Negative emotions that cause feelings of anger or dissatisfaction can disrupt beauty in the long term.

TCM can intervene by regulating the organs. A person who is prone to outbursts of anger is often manifesting the rising of liver heat. If the anger is more subdued and less apparent, or repressed, it may indicate a condition of liver stagnation. Both can be treated in TCM by different types of liver regulation.

Joy is the emotion related to the heart. Obviously a state of joy, as we conventionally think of it, is welcome by everyone. However "joy" can also encompass a state of excessive or constant excitement. An example of the negative effect of excess joy is lightheadedness or an attack of fainting that can sometimes actually be triggered by sudden good news.

Thinking is the mental activity related to the spleen. An excessive use of our thinking faculties, or over-thinking, and too much study may lead to stagnation or weakness of the spleen.

In other examples, sadness and worry on a long-term basis can easily weaken lung qi. Fear can cause kidney qi to sink down and the bladder to inefficiently hold urine. A deficiency of the kidney can often lead to a vicious cycle of more anxiety and fear.

Sound

Certain voice sounds and tones can be used in TCM diagnosis.

For example if someone tends to shout a lot in anger, it indicates an imbalance in the liver system. If someone laughs a lot without apparent reason, it indicates an imbalance in the heart system. A singing tone at inappropriate times and places can indicate an imbalance in the spleen system. Crying often may show a deficiency of the lung (whose emotion is grief). A very thin and weak voice also indicates weakness of lung qi. A groaning or husky tone of voice indicates an imbalance in the kidney system.

Tissues

Disharmony of the tissues, as defined by TCM, on a long-term basis can be used in diagnosis as a pointer to disharmony of the related organs. For instance if the tendons are tight and stiff, it may be because a liver or gallbladder disharmony exists. A problem with blood vessels points to a heart imbalance. A weakness or atrophy of the muscles indicates spleen deficiency. The skin is related to the lung, and a lung weakness often manifests with spontaneous sweating. The kidney is related to the bones and teeth, so teeth or bones that break easily or bone degenerative disorders that occur in old age, such as osteoporosis, are often due to the decline of kidney essence.

Sense Organs

Clinically, problems with the five senses can also reflect disharmonies in the relevant organs. For example blurred vision often reflects liver deficiency. A problem with the tongue can be related to the heart. Mouth and lips problems are often due to spleen deficiency or stomach heat. A dry nose and sneezing reflect lack of nourishment in the lung, while a decrease in hearing or chronic tinnitus can be due to kidney deficiency.

External Point of Appearance

We can also look to exterior manifestations in the nails, face, lips, body hair or scalp hair for information about disharmonies in related organs. If the liver is disordered, the nails of both the fingers and toes will be soft or deformed. If the heart is unbalanced, qi and blood will be disturbed, and facial complexion will be changed. If the spleen is unbalanced then pale, cracked or lusterless lips may be apparent. If the lung is disordered, body hair will appear withered. If the kidney is unbalanced, hair loss or color change might occur.

Liquids

Clinically, eyes that are sensitive (to wind or light) or that are constantly teary can be related to liver dysfunction. Emotional or nervous sweating is often due to heart weakness. Thin saliva that easily drips out when sleeping can indicate a spleen deficiency. Runny, clear nasal liquid can be related to a decline in the function of the lung. A chronic lack of thick saliva in the mouth, which is apparent in someone who has difficulty talking for long periods of time without the need for water, can indicate a kidney weakness.

5. Integrated Organ Systems

The relationships described above only partly tell the story. We need a combination of system markers to judge whether an imbalance can be related to other organs.

Besides the special system of *zang-fu* organ pairings described earlier, all internal organs need to be harmonized with each other as they interrelate to produce good quality blood, qi and body fluid. There are various types of relationships. These include "generation", like a mother and child relationship, which exists, for example, between the liver and heart. A relationship may also be one of "control" or "restriction", such as that between

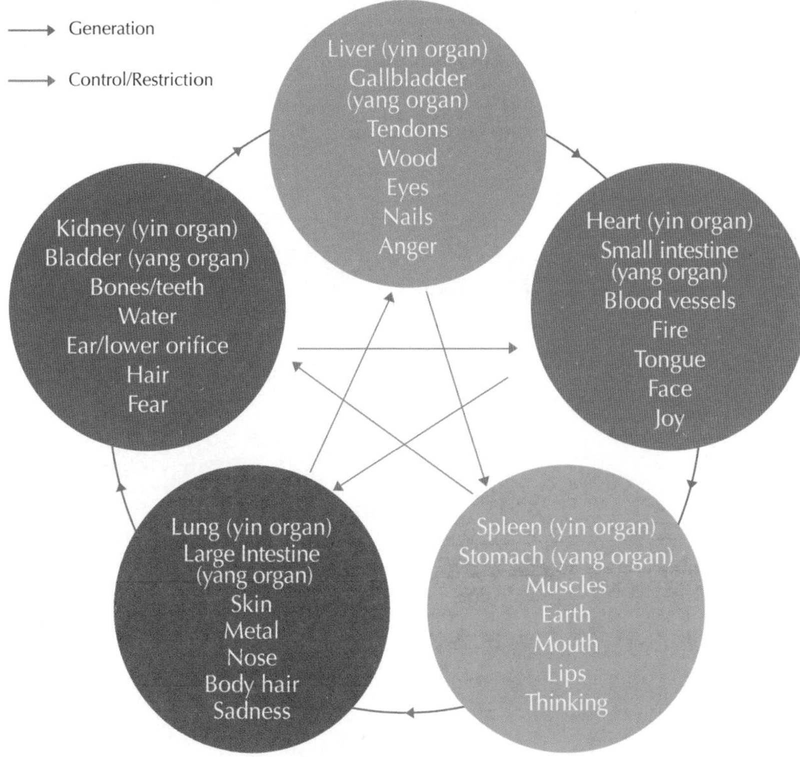

Fig. 6 Relationship between the organ systems

the liver and spleen (fig. 6).

Zang-fu organs also give each other a helping hand when in need. For instance if heart energy is weak, then the liver system can help to overcome this. Each organ system needs to work with the others, and they all need to be equally strong and functioning optimally in order to achieve robust health.

In upcoming chapters you will discover just how powerful these organ systems are in creating radiant beauty. Even without these details, it is clear that if you want to enhance beauty and maintain an ideal body, you need to look after the internal organ systems and foster a harmonious relationship between them. It is vital for the exterior that there is good inner circulating qi, nourished blood, and balanced yin and yang. All of these elements are carried by the meridians to make your body strong and flexible and to regulate your organs.

6. Qi, Blood, Body Fluid and the Organ Systems

Qi, blood and body fluid complement each other and have multifaceted relationships with the internal organ systems.

Qi has the function of promoting blood and body fluid circulation and metabolism, warming and protecting the body, and holding body liquid materials and internal organs in place. It also is responsible for aiding the transformation of nutrition, essence, blood and body fluids into one another. The kidney, spleen and lung are important for the production of qi.

Blood is inseparable from qi, and qi infuses life into blood. However blood is much denser and unlike qi cannot change into an invisible form. The spleen, lung, heart and kidney organ systems are vital for the production of blood.

Body fluids are called *jin ye* in Chinese. This word is composed of two characters, the first meaning "moist" or "saliva", which indicates anything that is liquid, and the second meaning "fluid", indicating fluids contained in living organisms (i.e. that found in vegetables and fruit). The stomach, spleen, small intestine and large intestine are necessary for the production of body fluids.

Dr. Fei Boxiong, a classically trained scholar and famous physician from the Qi dynasty noted the importance of these interrelationships: "Five *zang* and six *fu* organs produce qi and blood; when qi and blood are full of vigor, they nourish the *zang-fu* organs."

7. External Factors Influencing the Organ Systems

Another interesting concept integral to Chinese medicine is the fact that your organ systems are influenced by external factors, including the seasons and the time of day. The energy of each organ can change during the day, month, season and year.

In TCM we talk about the five seasons, adding to the traditional four seasons a rainy season, typically between summer and autumn. Your body adapts to the seasons, and changes occur in the body's functions according to the environment. For example spring is the season for germination, and is warm and windy. During summer, growth occurs and heat abounds. This is true in the body as well as externally. Transformation takes place during the rainy season but this season is damp. Autumn is a time for reaping and is dry, while winter is cold and is a season for storage.

If we focus on one season, we will see a variety of changes happening within the body. Winter is the time for preservation and conservation, and the slowdown of growth in winter can be observed in the external environment as well as the micro-environment of the body. For example, trees lose their leaves or slow down growth and animals go into hibernation.

Within your own body, in winter, you have less color in your face and your pulse rate is slower and deeper, because the blood vessels are deeper and more contracted in the colder seasons. Additionally your hair and nails will grow at a less rapid pace and your skin might become more rough and dry. Your pores will close and sweating will cease (for most people). This occurs to preserve your essence and to keep heat inside your body. During winter your body is prioritizing your organs. It is conserving energy and ensuring that your internal organs have enough yang qi.

Additionally your digestive function increases in winter, so you are able to take in more calories to help sustain the energy demands of the body, whereas in summer it reduces and you might not feel as hungry. Your body adapts intelligently to its environment.

The body also responds to the time of day. You may have heard of the TCM body clock, which describes the specific two-hour periods during a 24-hour period when each meridian is most active (fig. 7).

For instance, the time for the paired *zang-fu* organs of the gallbladder and liver is between 11 p.m. and 3 a.m. During this time the gallbladder and liver are re-harmonizing and detoxifying. This process is crucial for beauty sleep. It is also the best time for the metabolism to readjust, and since the liver helps the other organs to detoxify, this time is an essential time for resting your body. Your gallbladder is most active between 11 p.m. to 1 a.m., so it is important to be asleep at this time.

The stomach's peak time is between 7 a.m. and 9 a.m., so your digestive fire (as defined in TCM) is strongest at this time. Since assimilation of nutrients is most effective between these hours, it is essential to eat a nourishing breakfast during this time in order to boost your energy for the day.

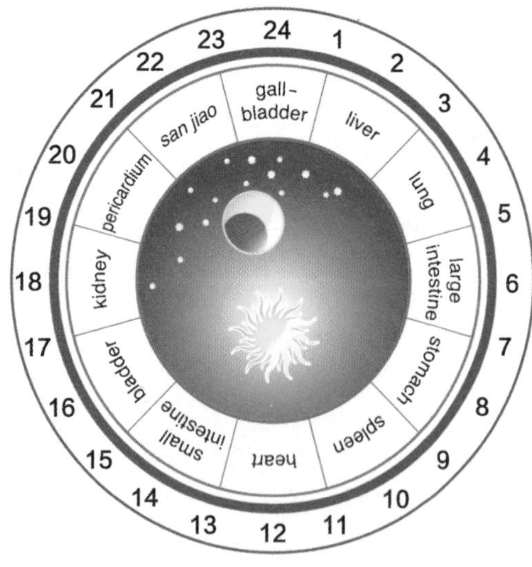

Fig. 7 TCM body clock

TCM 24-hour Body Clock			
Chinese Time	**Time**	**Meridian in Its Prime**	**Organ System**
Zi Time	11 p.m. to 1 a.m.	Gallbladder meridian	Liver system
Chou Time	1 a.m. to 3 a.m.	Liver meridian	
Yin Time	3 a.m. to 5 a.m.	Lung meridian	Lung system
Mao Time	5 a.m. to 7 a.m.	Large intestine meridian	
Chen Time	7 a.m. to 9 a.m.	Stomach meridian	Spleen system
Si Time	9 a.m. to 11 a.m.	Spleen meridian	
Wu Time	11 a.m. to 1 p.m.	Heart meridian	Heart system
Wei Time	1 p.m. to 3 p.m.	Small intestine meridian	
Shen Time	3 p.m. to 5 p.m.	Bladder meridian	Kidney system
You Time	5 p.m. to 7 p.m.	Kidney meridian	
Xu Time	7 p.m. to 9 p.m.	Pericardium meridian	Heart system
Hai Time	9 p.m. to 11 p.m.	*San jiao* meridian	

These are just a few examples of how your organs are affected by the time of day, and how you can work with your body to support their functions. Furthermore, throughout the course of a season, the energy of specific organs may fluctuate. So if you are aware of this, you can learn to work in harmony with the cycle of peaks and lows—getting more done during peaks and taking it easier during the low energy times.

CHAPTER TWO

Beauty from the Inside Out

Now that we know more about the Chinese belief, *yi nei yang wai*, or nourish the inside so it shines outwardly, we can see that a beautiful appearance is achievable only if one is truly healthy. Beauty is an "inside job", meaning that beauty is created on a cellular level and manifests in a healthy body and radiant complexion.

In this chapter we will discover how each organ system affects your appearance in various ways, and how they work together to impact your skin, hair, eyes and figure. Beauty issues can often be traced back to one or two organ systems. However this is not always the case, and sometimes they can be caused by other organs as well. Here we will use a three-star system to show the relevance between aspects of beauty and the organ systems:

★★★ High-level relevance

★★☆ Mid-level relevance

★☆☆ Low-level relevance

To treat the beauty issue, you should treat the high-level relevance organ first. If you are not getting the results you hope for after treatment, you can then investigate what else may be going on.

Relationships between Beauty and Internal Organs					
	Heart	Liver	Spleen	Lung	Kidney
Skin (including face and body skin)	★★☆	★☆☆	★★☆	★★★	★☆☆
Hair (including scalp, pubic and armpit hair, eyebrows and eyelashes)	★☆☆	★★☆	★☆☆	★★☆	★★★
Eyes	★★☆	★★★	★☆☆	★★☆	★☆☆
Body shape and build	★☆☆	★★☆	★★★	★☆☆	★★☆

1. Skin

When we refer to skin, we are referring to the skin's surface, sweat glands, body hair and other relevant tissues. Skin has four functions:

- Provide a protective surface to defend the internal body against external factors.
- Help regulate the metabolism of water. When sweating, your secrete water through your skin.
- Help stabilize body temperature. Since the skin covers the entire body, it is effective in letting excess heat out. During fever, exercise or summer, you may notice that you are sweating a lot. This is your body's way of regulating body temperature. Even when you cannot see visible sweat, you are constantly eliminating waste through the skin pores.
- Help with respiration. Skin can breathe, and this function is important to the overall oxygen level in your body according to Chinese medicine. Your sweat pores can be referred to as the "doors of qi".

Conditions such as pimples, inflammation and eczema are all indications that something is out of balance internally. Skin issues can often be traced back to the lung organ system. Treatment for skin conditions will often be a combined approach of treating the lung system along with other organs that are contributing to the problem. Radiant skin is created as a result of all of the organ systems working in harmony and coordinating well.

Lung and Skin ★★★

From the skin's function, it is obvious that lung and skin are closely related:

- First, the lung warm and nourish the skin. The dispersing function of the lung aids in spreading body fluid and defensive qi to the skin. When the skin and body hair are nourished adequately by body fluid and defensive qi, the skin will have luster and hair will be glossy.
- Second, the lung insure the security of the body surface. As defensive qi flows under the skin, it assists in resisting exterior pathogenic factors. If lung qi is weak, defensive qi will also be weak. This will cause spontaneous sweating. Over time, excess sweating can result in the loss of a certain amount of defensive qi, leaving the person prone to attacks by exterior pathogenic factors. If a pathogen does invade the exterior of the body, for instance the skin and muscles, it may obstruct the skin pores and disturb the function of the lung and defensive qi. Symptoms may arise such as a runny nose, cough or lung disorder.
- Third, the lung regulate skin function. The lung can control the opening and closing of the skin pores, regulating the temperature of body and further influencing the appearance of the skin.
- Fourth, the skin and body hair assist the lung in regulating respiratory function. The opening and closing of the pores help to scatter lung qi and to regulate respiration and assist in excreting waste.

If the above functions are impaired, the skin may be rough

and dry, and the body hair may be withered. In Chapter Eight, we will discuss the relationship between the lung and the skin in more detail and provide some solutions.

Heart and Skin ★★☆

The heart organ system is responsible for managing your blood, blood circulation and vessels. It also controls the spiritual element of your being.

Obviously the heart needs a good amount of blood to nourish the amazing skin that covers your entire body. This blood flow is important in delivering nutrients to every cell. Ensuring that blood moves smoothly in the vessels is another responsibility of the heart, so enlarged veins or spider veins visible through the skin are linked back to this organ.

Since the heart governs your spirit and mind, and the heart corresponds to summer, skin issues that only occur at night and during summer can often be linked to the heart system. Skin itchiness and dryness during sleep, or skin rash in summer may be addressed by balancing the heart. During the night your heart helps to foster sound sleep and feelings of well-being. It also works at harmonizing all the yin and yang in your body. These factors contribute toward calm sleep and lovely glowing skin. If heart blood and yin are not strong enough, skin issues such as pimples, summer rash and boils can occur.

Spleen and Skin ★★☆

Cou li, meaning the skin texture and fascia between the muscles, is very important in TCM. It was believed that original qi and body fluids are metabolized in this area.

Since the spleen controls the muscles, the lung need to cooperate with the spleen to make the *cou li* healthy. The lung ensure that defensive qi performs its function of opening and closing the skin pores, which is vital for protection. The lung and spleen create elasticity, softness and smoothness in the skin and allow it to hold moisture.

Hydrated skin mainly comes from the inside, and has very little to do with what kind of product you put on the skin surface. It is quite common in China for women to just wash their faces and never, or rarely, apply moisturizer. Many 80-year-olds have enviable skin that rivals their daughter's, and a glow to their complexion without the need for expensive products. Some of these women even use special herbal and nourishing soups to create beautiful skin.

Liver and Skin ★☆☆

The role of the liver is to store blood, so it is quite important for your skin. If the liver is healthy, it can store enough blood and send it to all areas of the body as needed.

If you can release your stress and deal with anger promptly, your skin will experience better blood circulation and receive more nutrients. Chronic anger can lead to liver stagnation resulting in a breakout of pimples.

Stagnation of the liver can show up on your face. Some women experience a little bit of acne or a few pimples prior to menstruation; this is also linked to the liver. Liver energy should be evenly spread around the body, but when the uterus holds a lot of blood (just prior to menstruation) and the breasts and abdominal region become a little full (in preparation in case a women becomes pregnant), sometimes the liver can struggle to distribute qi around the body. This is often made worse by eating a lot of hot, spicy food and having a great deal of stress. These small blockages of energy might manifest on the face and back in the form of pimples. This is why when menstruation arrives, pimples usually disappear. After menstruation all the liver anger and stagnation can leave the body through the blood, and the liver qi can flow smoothly once again.

Pregnancy pigmentation can also be traced back to the liver. Pregnancy is a healthy kind of "blockage", and some of the stagnated energy might cause pigmentation to appear on the skin. This type of pigmentation can sometimes disappear on its own after pregnancy, but can also be cleared by nourishing the liver and blood during the first three months post-partum. Failing to nourish the liver and blood may cause the pigmentation to become permanent. Varicose veins during pregnancy can also be linked to a stagnation of energy.

Kidney and Skin ★☆☆

Since the kidney organ stores congenital essence and contributes to DNA, according to TCM, the appearance of your skin, in part, is influenced by your ethnic and genetic inheritance.

At the same time, radiant skin that lasts a lifetime is dependent upon kidney function. On a short-term basis, you can derive nourishment from the foods and liquids you consume daily, and your kidney will help with the storage of essence derived from these nutrients. But in your 70s, digestive capability becomes weaker, so your body begins to rely on stored essence for long-lasting beautiful skin. A good supply of stored essence will help to prevent saggy, dry skin and keep wrinkles at bay. The essence stored by the kidney consists of two parts, congenital (from your parents) and acquired (from the essential substances of food), which help and rely on each other.

Some skin conditions can be linked to imbalances in the kidney system. Disturbances in color metabolism, such as vitiligo, can have a genetic component. Treatment in the earlier stages seems to be most effective, and the condition can be reversed or at least halted if it is dealt with quickly. In some extreme cases, preventing the spread of this condition can be achieved, but a skin graft is used to cover the existing patches.

Another condition that may have a genetic component is

eczema. It is further exasperated by too much dampness mixed with heat, or too much dryness mixed with dampness. As eczema further develops there are often large areas of skin that are dry; however dampness is coming into the body through the skin or diet. When this condition is present, foods that cause dampness should be limited.

Psoriasis is another skin condition that is remedied by treating the kidney. In fact any chronic, complicated skin condition can be addressed by treating the lung in combination with the kidney. This is because according to Five Elements Theory, the kidney and lung are "mother" and "child" in relationship.

Twelve Skin Zones

The surface skin of your face and body is divided into twelve zones, which are related to your twelve meridians. By noticing issues or problems within a specific zone, it is possible to figure out which organ system may out of balance (fig. 8).

Additional Factors Influencing Skin

Even if diet is similar in different locations, the environmental differences will have an impact on skin conditions. Your skin is affected by factors such as too much sun, wind and harsh environments.

For instance, in general, those living in Shanghai have a different quality to their skin than those living in Beijing. Shanghai is quite humid while Beijing is drier and has a lot of windstorms, which can strip the skin of moisture.

Organ's Preference for Environment

Kidney		Cold
Liver		Wind
Lung	Dislikes	Dryness
Spleen		Dampness
Heart		Heat

It is helpful to know the preferences each

Fig. 8 Skin Zones and the Related Meridians

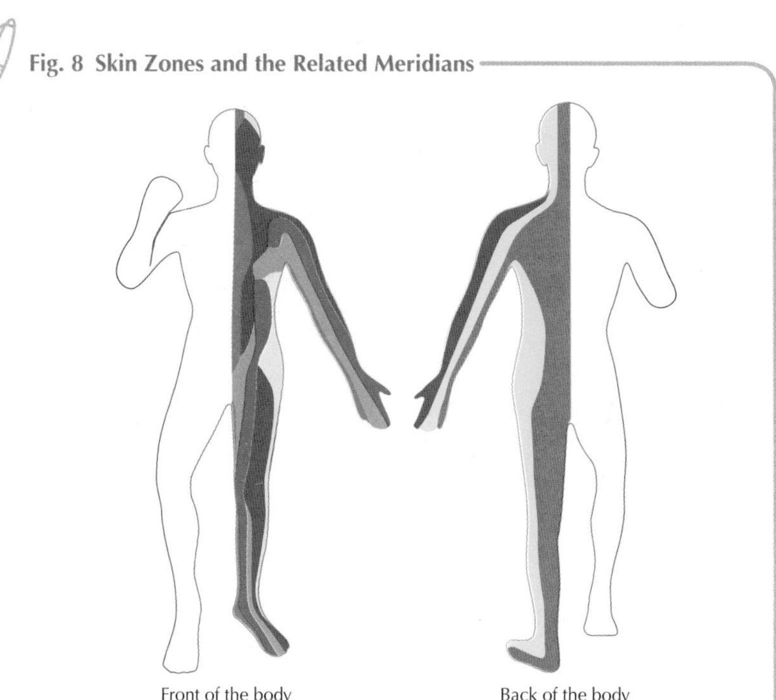

Color of Skin Zone	Sub-Category	Meridian	Treats
	Taiyang	Bladder Meridian of Foot	Kidney system
		Small Intestine Meridian of Hand	Heart system
	Yangming	Large Intestine Meridian of Hand	Lung system
		Stomach Meridian of Foot	Spleen system
	Shaoyang	Gallbladder Meridian of Foot	Liver system
		San Jiao Meridian of Hand	Heart system
	Taiyin	Lung Meridian of Hand	Lung system
		Spleen Meridian of Foot	Spleen system
	Shaoyin	Heart Meridian of Hand	Heart system
		Kidney Meridian of Foot	Kidney system
	Jueyin	Liver Meridian of Foot	Liver system
		Pericardium Meridian of Hand	Heart system

organ has for certain environments. With this in mind, you can make dietary choices to counteract environmental elements. In China people may eat foods that moisten the lung before autumn (because autumn is dry), warming foods before winter, foods that clear dampness before times of high humidity, and cool foods to protect against heat before summer.

For instance you may notice patches of dryness, varicose or spider veins, or pigmentation in certain regions. Taking note of where these conditions regularly appear can help with diagnosis. You can use the "twelve skin zone" theory as a reference tool. A TCM practitioner might treat the meridians related to these zones with acupuncture, massage and acupressure.

The heart system controls the meridians of the heart, small intestine, pericardium and *san jiao*. According this theory, if a skin condition is found in any of these areas you might look at treating the heart system first. Likewise for the other systems: The lung system controls the lung and large intestine zones. The liver system controls the liver and gallbladder zones. The spleen system controls the spleen and stomach zones, while the kidney system controls the kidney and bladder zones.

Tips

To review, for any type of skin condition, it is important to first look to the lung and see if the lung system needs support. Take measures to prevent environmental dryness from impacting your lung system. Deal with your sadness and worries rather than allowing them to consume your life. Chronic sadness can drag your facial muscles down so try to smile more often to strengthen the muscles that lift your face upward.

Secondly, use the self-assessment in Chapter Four to analyze which organ or organ systems may need additional support. Use this along with the twelve skin zones map to see which organ systems may need the application of food or herbal remedies, acupuncture or changes in lifestyle.

Thirdly, pay attention to cold, heat, dryness and dampness in your body. Also consider the season and environment when planning and fine-tuning your diet. For instance, if you live in an area that is very dry, you might do something to counteract it and balance the dryness, like consuming wolfberries (goji berries, *gou qi*). In China people eat a lot of lily bulb (in food and drink), tremella (also known as silver ear or white fungus), pears and avocado in autumn and winter, to counteract the dryness of the environment. These foods nourish the lung and protect against dryness. In Beijing, they might consume these foods more often than in Shanghai, due to the fact that Beijing is drier.

It is a good habit to tonify the organ before the season begins; in this way Chinese people plan their diet a season in advance, taking special care to include foods that help to balance the effects of the coming season. In winter, foods and tonics that protect against cold, such as animal products, are often valued. Since the digestive system is more active during winter, your body can digest these foods more effectively during these months. Since people are a bit more inactive in winter and sleep longer, this nourishment consumed is easily stored as essence instead of being used. These are general guidelines, but it is always important to listen to the needs of your individual constitution.

2. Hair

In this section "hair" refers to the hair on the head. There are many Chinese traditional and cultural beliefs regarding hair. For example, boys are thought to be more yang in character and therefore their hair should also be more vigorous. If a young boy develops thin, fine hair in his early years, the parents will often shave it all off to stimulate hair growth. Since girls are more yin in nature, parents often don't mind if their hair is soft and fine when they are little. However if they don't have much hair growth over a period of a year their parents might also cut it short.

Furthermore, in China, if an adult has lost a lot of hair they will often cut it and keep it short for a period of time while they take herbs to tonify their essence and blood. Afterward hair might be grown long again.

Often, professional people who work in jobs that require a lot of thinking have short hair. This tradition comes from the belief that thinking and stress require a great deal of kidney essence and blood; your brain also needs both these substances especially in jobs that demand a lot of mental work. Cutting the hair allows one to re-strengthen the organ systems.

Your genetics have a say in the color of your hair, and how fine or thick it is. How oily or dry your hair is also can depend on genetics, how often you wash it, and also on the type of foods you regularly consume. But at the same time, the concept that the hair is an extension of your blood is important in TCM, so any organ system involved in creating and distributing blood will also influence the growth, texture, shine and hydration of your hair.

Kidney and Hair ★★★

The kidney strengthens the hair through the transformation of essence into blood. Additionally, congenital kidney essence also ensures that the color, growth and quantity of hair is optimal. Voluminous and soft hair that has depth in its color is highly valued, and it is not possible without a healthy kidney system.

Your hair relies on nourishment from your kidney essence. If kidney essence is abundant, the hair will grow well and be healthy and glossy. If kidney essence is weak or declining, the hair will become thin, brittle, dull-looking and grey.

In childhood, kidney essence develops, and hair grows longer and faster. During youth and middle age, kidney essence flourishes, and the hair is lustrous and rich in color. As one ages, this essence declines and the hair turns dry, grey and falls out. These are normal physiological condition in life. But for abnormalities—hair that grows slowly, thinly or not at all in childhood, premature grey hair, or losing hair too rapidly—we have answers in TCM.

So in short, to maintain beautiful hair, TCM pays special attention to the kidney system.

Liver and Hair ★★☆

The hair is very much influenced by the liver, because the liver organ stores blood and ensures that qi flows effectively throughout the entire body. Hair needs a lot of blood and qi to grow.

The liver's role in regulating emotions is also an important factor in keeping hair healthy. Negative emotions can lead to liver stagnation. If liver qi becomes chronically stagnated, the blood will be unable to ascend to your hair effectively. This stagnated energy can get stuck in the midsection rather than circulating to the rest of the body. Stress can play a role in hair loss, so keeping the liver strong, which ensures a higher tolerance to stress, will result in keeping the liver free from stagnation.

Furthermore, managing your emotions will promote sounder sleep. If people with a strong liver have stressful jobs, they can step back from the situation, rest and deal with the issue from a fresh perspective rather than allowing it to affect their emotions and sleep patterns. Those who are unable to escape from stressful events may not be able to regulate their emotions and may have more hair loss.

So we can see that tonifying the liver's blood and regulating emotions can help you grow thick, shiny hair.

Lung and Hair ★★☆

A strong, well-functioning lung system will also contribute toward lovely hair. The lung has an important job to do, ensuring that energy is ascending and descending effectively throughout your body.

The ascending feature is particularly important for the hair because it will ensure that qi, blood and body fluids are adequately reaching the skin surface and rising to the top of the head. This helps hair grow.

The season of the lung is autumn according to Five Elements Theory. During autumn it is natural for people to experience some hair loss. It can be likened to trees that lose their leaves in autumn and regenerate themselves in spring. While some hair loss is normal, if it is excessive, this could be caused by dehydrated lung that cannot tolerant dryness in autumn.

You can take measures to prevent hair loss if you strengthen and nourish the lung and kidney during autumn. It is important to also focus on the kidney since the lung is the "mother" of the kidney in Five Elements Theory.

Spleen and Hair ★☆☆

The spleen organ is also relevant to the health of your hair to some extent. It transforms and transports the food and liquids you consume, ensuring a good quantity and quality of blood and qi for daily use.

It has often been noted that children who have a weak digestive system or spleen weakness may have less hair as well as dullness of hair color.

It is good to note the darkest color your hair has ever been naturally (without dye); the depth and richness of this color is likely to be your natural hair color. If your hair begins to lighten and become thinner, it could be because of a spleen imbalance. Oily hair and dandruff can also be related to the spleen, indicating that it has been blocked by dampness.

You should take special note of other markers of spleen disharmony, and if necessary, support your digestion and spleen system. The spleen is the root of the qi and blood in the body and it also prevents blood from "leaking". Therefore if your spleen is functioning well, you will have clear, yang energy flowing to your head as well as blood flow to your hair ensuring that it is nourished and hydrated, without accumulating dampness.

Heart and Hair ★☆☆

By transforming body fluids and nutrition qi into red blood, your heart organ keeps you alive and nourishes every cell in your body. The color of the heart in Five Elements Theory is red and it has special yang energy. Even if you have enough body fluid and nutrition qi, if your heart system is not strong you may not create enough blood. Yang is vital for producing healthy blood.

The heart controls the blood and the blood vessels to ensure good circulation, which is needed for hair. The heart is the "emperor" of the whole organ system, and problems with the system manifest in many ways. Insomnia, dream disturbance, feeling constantly annoyed and anxious, heart palpitations, poor sleep quality, being quick to take offense, and chest pains can all be indications that your heart needs some support. Unfortunately it will also mean that you are more susceptible to hair loss and grey hair, as the lack of blood circulation or deficiency of blood can significantly impact blood flow to the head. When the blood of the heart is insufficient the hair will be affected.

Tips

Those who wish to have long hair should tonify their blood from time to time with certain foods, including wolfberries, jujubes (Chinese dates) and iron-rich foods such as wood ear (black fungus, *hei mu er*), beetroot and spinach.

Whether your hair ends becomes split or remains resistant to splitting depends on how easy it is for blood to spread equally to all areas of your body including the hair. If you have a lot of split ends, it indicates your kidney energy can only support its growth to a particular length at that point in time.

Hair loss can occur more frequently when sleeping patterns or emotions become unbalanced. Stress, sleep disorders and strong emotions can take their toll on your hair. If you are starting to notice a receding hairline, try to go to sleep earlier, no later than 10:30 or 11 pm on most nights.

Greying in patches, slow growth or lack of growth can all be remedied with TCM, and it is possible to delay hair loss and greying in both men and women, especially if it is addressed early. Adding a hair massage routine and balancing or tonifying the organs can also work wonders.

3. Eyes

Many organs contribute to the appearance and health of the eyes, and the eyes can reveal much about each organ system. The Han dynasty TCM classic, *Spiritual Axis* (*Ling Shu Jing*) says: "The essence of the five yin and the six yang organs ascends to the eyes."

There are certain regions of the eyes that refer to specific organ systems (fig. 9):

- Iris: Different ethnicities may have different iris colors. For example in general Asians have dark brown irises while Western European usually have blue or light brown irises. The brightness or darkness of the environment can change the size of iris. Since the liver controls the free movement of energy, the iris belongs to the liver system.
- Blood vessels: The color red and the blood vessels have close relationships with the heart, therefore both the inner corner (pink/red colored flesh) and outer corner (capillary) of the eyes belong to the heart.
- Eyelid: The function and strength of the muscles come from

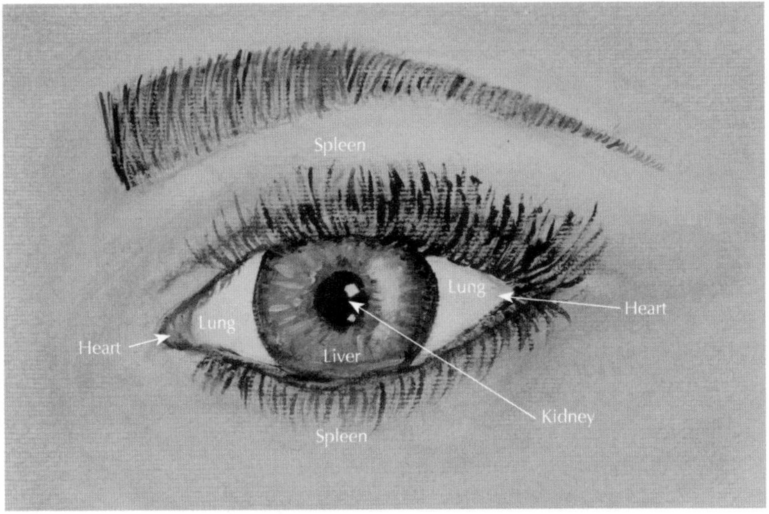

Fig. 9 The eye map

energy and nourishment of the spleen. So the eyelids are more related to the spleen.

- Whites: In the Five Elements color system, the color while pairs with lung. So the whites of the eyes belong to the lung.
- Pupil: There is eye fluid from the back of the eye through pupil to front of the eye, in order to balance water metabolism of the eyes. The kidney governs water, so the pupil belong to the kidney.

Therefore if you constantly notice a particular region of the eye is experiencing some type of dysfunction, you should investigate whether the organ related to that section is out of balance.

Liver and Eyes ★★★

According to the Five Elements Theory, the liver belongs to the element of wood, and the liver system "opens up" in your eyes.

The liver stores blood and ensures the smooth flow of qi.

Liver qi draws liver blood up into the eyes to provide nourishment for the eyes. Well-nourished eyes have good vision and are able to identify different colors. If liver blood is abundant, the eyes will be adequately moist and vision will be sharp. If liver blood is weak, there may be blurred vision, myopia, "floaters" in the eyes or color blindness, or the eyes may feel dry and gritty.

The liver also regulates the body's energy. This is important for the production of body fluids, including tears to moisten and protect the eyes. Another reason the health of the liver impacts the eyes is due to the liver meridian. The Jueyin Liver Meridian of Foot is directly linked to the eye system, superficially as well as deep inside. It helps to regulate the entire eye system, including the metabolism of water and blood.

Sour fruits and the color green are nourishing, especially in spring. Being surrounded by green, as one would be in nature, is beneficial for the liver, and it relaxes the eyes and helps them feel rested.

Heart and Eyes ★★☆

TCM draws upon four different diagnostic methods to diagnose illness. These include looking, hearing, inquiry and touch. Looking into the eyes can prove to be a powerful diagnostic tool.

Harmony between the physical body and the mind can be observed in the eyes. A person's mental focus and energy will show in the eyes. If the eyes are clear and sparkle, they indicate a good state of mind. Thus the fundamental TCM classic *Yellow Emperor's Canon* (*Huang Di Nei Jing*) described the eyes as the outer representation of the heart as they provide a window into the soul (fig. 10).

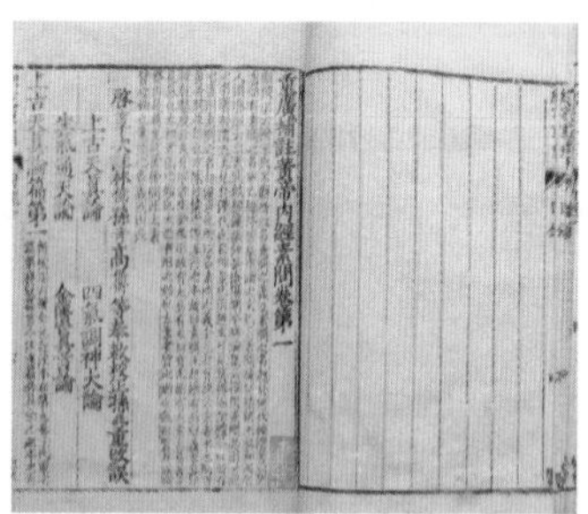

Fig. 10 *Yellow Emperor's Canon* is a classic of TCM.

There are many blood vessels linking to the back of the eyes. If these blood vessels do not receive good blood circulation then vision might become compromised. If the corners of the eyes are red, treat the heart first.

Lung and Eyes ★★☆

The lung is responsible for governing qi. The production of qi and the function of directing qi movement throughout your entire body is dependent upon a healthy lung system and quality breathing.

We have learned that blood follows qi. So if you have a lack of qi or qi stagnation, your eyes will not receive the blood flow or nutrition they need. Then your vision may be affected, including an inability to focus or see clearly. Meditation, relaxation and breathing exercises help to increase qi and facilitate better qi movement, leading to better eyesight. Research shows that people who partake in outdoor activities have better vision.

Efficient and smooth water metabolism is influenced by the descending and ascending functions of the lung. This is also important for the eyes. The ascending function ensures that clean water can come up to the eyes, and the descending function sends wastewater down to the lower orifices. Furthermore, in the early stage of exposure to an illness, bacteria or virus, the lung's defensive qi will help protect the eyes from outside factors.

Spleen and Eyes ★☆☆

The spleen governs the muscles, including the muscles of the upper and lower eyelids. Strength of vision and the ability to avoid eye fatigue depend on how much nutrition can reach the muscles around the eyes.

Soreness after using your eyes for a short time and a feeling of fullness in the eyes can be linked to suboptimal spleen function. Sleeping with the eyes half open is another tell-tale sign that the spleen is not controlling the eye muscles effectively.

Bloodshot eyes, when there is no infection present, is an

indication that the spleen is not effectively keeping the blood in the blood vessels, causing blood to leak into the eye system. With this condition, there is also a lack of good circulation. Bags under the eyes, including big ones that form during middle age, as well as early morning puffiness, may be communicating that you need to balance and strengthen spleen function.

Kidney and Eyes ★☆☆

Vision problems can be caused by a variety of factors, which include vitamin or mineral deficiencies, and swelling of the eyeballs and eye muscles due to overuse, especially when we study or stare at computer screens too long without periods of rest. Some degenerative conditions of the eyes can be an age-related process, and can be linked back to the kidney system.

Kidney essence is important to your health and longevity, as it can transform into qi and blood. Essence, qi and blood are vital substances that nourish your eyes. Kidney essence can protect your eyes against blurred or distorted vision, and it also helps you to identify colors.

In TCM the eye system is attached to brain marrow. Healthy marrow, nourished by the kidney, is important for the eye system, and clear pupils indicate healthy marrow. According to *Yellow Emperor's Canon*, weak kidney essence can lead to the shrinkage of brain marrow, which may cause dizziness, tinnitus and blurred vision. If the marrow is not functioning properly or shrinks, or if there is a blood blockage, this can disturb vision significantly.

A swelling or black color under the eyes indicates kidney deficiency.

Tips

Beautiful eyes require a healthy liver system, first and foremost. Traditionally, in China, people take measures to ensure that the liver has enough blood and that liver qi makes its way to the eyes.

Furthermore in keeping all your organ systems healthy, they can symbiotically work together to create healthy eyes.

These steps will help you achieve optimal eye function:

- Avoid liver fire or stagnation to keep great vision.
- Avoid getting angry too often; try to keep a happy and positive mental state, reducing negative emotions.
- Get enough sleep to improve vision.
- Have a broad range of interests and let your inner beauty shine forth.
- Engage with others and take time to rest your eyes. Participate in sports and outdoor exercise. Encourage your children to go out and play rather than looking at electronic devices for hours on end.
- TCM eye massage and resting eyes with a warm cloth over them can help strengthen weak vision.

4. Body Shape

The impact that the organs have on body shape is often not given enough credence. Their combined efforts keep your figure balanced and strong:

- The spleen transforms food into energy, and ensures that your muscles receive enough energy and blood. It also ensures that the limbs are shapely.
- The liver stores blood and regulates the circulation of qi, so that you are able to have elastic, strong tendons and ligaments. This promotes flexibility and stability in the joints.
- The kidney nourishes bones and spinal marrow, which contribute to an upright framework and posture.
- The heart (the body's "emperor") also influences body shape and posture. When people are tired or have mental fatigue, maintaining an upright posture and good

circulation can become difficult. If someone is depressed, they will often slouch; if they are happy and positive, they are more likely to stand upright with open body language.

- The lung (the body's "prime minister") contributes to the body's energy. If one can't breathe well or can't discard waste through the skin, nose or mouth, the muscles and tendons will become weak because fresh energy cannot support their needs.

The body's growth and development are not only influenced by the effective functioning of the five organ systems, but also the state of the reproductive system. One's height and build have some genetic influences, but the reproductive system, specifically hormones, can also influence physical build. Healthy, balanced hormones are vital for an optimal body shape. Healthy organ systems will help to create balanced hormones.

So if you take care of the organ systems, you will be contributing toward the health of your bones, ligaments, tendons and muscles. At the same time, you will also be ensuring the natural changes that occur in your hormones throughout life happen smoothly and without issue.

You cannot change the genes you have inherited, but you can change how they are expressed. Balance and cooperation between the five organ systems will help you express the best and healthiest genes.

Spleen and Body Shape ★★★

We may look to the spleen to resolve a number of body issues relating to lifestyle changes. For example, after marriage one may gain a lot of weight or those who previously had dry skin may find their skin is oilier. This may be because of a different lifestyle after marriage, such as spend more time eating than exercising. There are many things that can be done: changing your eating pattern, eating different types of food, not eating a heavy dinner, and so on.

In China, there is a saying, "After food, walk 100 steps and you can live 99 years." This idea is good for digestion and easier than you might think. Of course you don't need to count out exactly 100 steps; moving in a relaxed way after eating can prevent the spleen from getting blocked by food and ultimately facilitates digestion. A person who cleans up will be less likely to gain as much weight as a person who just sits in front of the television after eating.

There are many Chinese supplements and food remedies that mainly target the spleen system. For instance, pearl barley is well known as a spleen-supporting food, and is used in China to promote shapely legs and arms. Many Chinese film stars consume pearl barley as a soup. Pearl barley is detoxifying, it helps to prevent lumps and polyps, and brings excess water out of the body through the urinary bladder. It is also a powerful tonic to reduce dampness.

Another food that can help reduce weight is bitter melon (*ku gua*), which is useful for helping the spleen get rid of dampness. Scientific studies have also shown that lentils can be beneficial for reducing weight and the size of the stomach.

Tummy breathing and holding energy in that region can also lift the stomach and help with muscle tone.

Liver and Body Shape ★★☆

As we have learned, the liver regulates emotions. A weak liver will weaken your tolerance for different kinds of emotions, potentially causing emotional eating. Emotional eating will further weaken the liver, leading to a vicious cycle.

Try to deal with your emotions at the root cause rather than using the "sweet solution" to avoid facing the problem. Learning to balance your life with hobbies is also important. Eating a poor and unbalanced diet, binge eating, irregular meal times, eating snacks instead of meals, and eating more than you need, will all take a toll on the liver.

Getting enough exercise and keeping a good schedule can help to promote a balanced liver. Excess weight can easily creep on due to inactivity, so it is important to schedule exercise into your day.

Kidney and Body Shape ★★☆

The kidney is the administrative organ with the greatest power, as it is the congenital base of life and stores essence. The kidney acts as the strength and intelligence of the entire body, and is responsible for its overall constitution. It has a clear link to body shape, as it governs the body's growth and development as well as the maturation of the reproductive systems. While partly based on heredity, one's own health management also influences the kidney's overall state.

Some weight concerns start from puberty, while some appear during middle age or climacteric syndrome. One's build and weight are influenced by genetics, but the kidney's power in balancing yin and yang can reduce some hereditary influences.

As mentioned, the kidney controls the metabolism of body fluids, so the circulation of fluids within the body is influenced by the kidney. If kidney function is good, then the body will receive adequate fluids and remain free from blockages. Water retention in any one part of the body may influence overall fluid metabolism and its ability to nourish the body.

Water retention during your menstrual cycle can be addressed by supporting the liver and kidney. Since weight gain can also be caused by illnesses such as hypothyroid issues, strengthening kidney function can control and slow down the development of the disease.

Tips for Gaining Weight

Some people become underweight after an operation or illness, while some are born with a weak digestive system or have certain intolerances or allergies. It is important to investigate and find the cause of your own situation. If there is an underlying intolerance or allergy, then you must address this root cause. Supporting the digestive system is often necessary in order to regain weight. If you have chronic diarrhea it may be hard to gain weight, so you must find the cause and address it.

The treatment depends on the situation. For those with a picky appetite, one must treat the stomach to open the appetite. Those with an appetite but difficulty digesting food may have a spleen or gallbladder deficiency. These conditions may cause loose stools or discomfort in the abdominal region. If the gallbladder is the culprit, then a bitter taste might be present in the mouth, or there may be an aversion to oily or fatty food. If the spleen is to blame, then bloating might occur in the belly button region, accompanied by a heavy and lethargic mind. The mouth may crave strong tastes while the taste may be dull.

In TCM clinical practice, in order to facilitate weight gain or to support weak digestion, we would try to warm the spleen. When the spleen is deficient in fire, qi and yang, it can impair digestion. The stomach needs "digestive fire" to effectively break down food. If your digestive system is too cold, due to yang deficiency from the heart or kidney, then you may have trouble with digestion. In this case adjusting the spleen alone may not be effective. Using yang tonics to warm the heart and kidney will help to provide yang energy for the spleen.

Five-spice and rosemary can be effective yang tonics for the heart. Rosemary also goes to the twelve meridians, or "energy highways", and people often use it during winter or cook it with lamb, which is also warming (fig. 11). In general, warming, spicy foods function as yang tonics for the heart and kidney. Using a lot of ginger prepared with pork can warm a cold stomach.

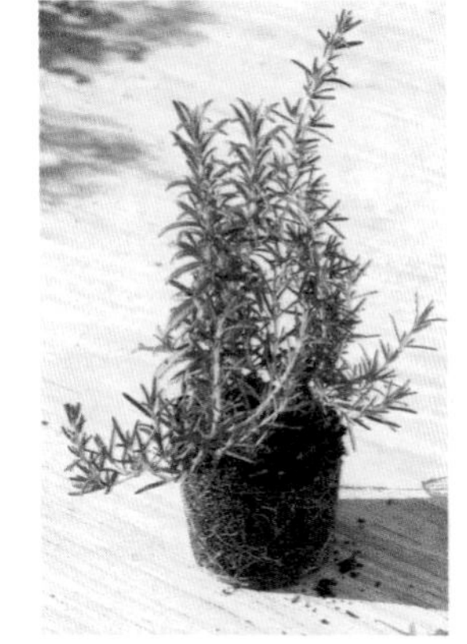
Fig. 11 Rosemary

It is common for people in China to

eat animal organs to strengthen their own organs. One special dish is a soup made with the stomach lining of a chicken. However if this is not a dish for you, then using ginger, five-spice, fresh fennel, cloves and star anise are good options. These spices are all excellent in helping to warm the body. Clove and cinnamon powder paste for external use is available in Chinese pharmacies.

Increased participation in sports, as well as just moving the arms and legs, will further promote beneficial stomach motion and support digestive and absorption functions.

Furthermore staying up all night and sleeping during the day are both not good for hormone balance, which can further influence weight.

Tips for Losing Weight

Firstly, evaluate how much food you need for the production of good nutrition, qi and body fluids, compared to how much energy you typically use. Those with labor intensive jobs may be able to afford to eat more than those who sit at a desk all day long.

Be sure to enjoy the food you eat and appreciate all the flavors and tastes. Eating foods that includes a balance of properties (such as hot, warm, cold and cool) and flavors (such as sweat, sour, salty,

Notice How You Feel Before and After Eatting

Q: Are you able to eat without symptoms of gas, bloating or burping?
A: This means you have chosen food that easy to digest and suits your constitution. Avoid foods that provoke intolerance and allergies. If you do experience any of the above symptoms, evaluate the kinds of food you are eating and whether they suit your body.
Q: Before a meal, do you feel hungry or are you just eating out of habit?
A: It is best to wait until you feel hungry.
Q: Do you feel lethargic after food?
A: If so, you may have eaten too much food or food that is too heavy. Eat only until you are 70% full.

spicy and bitter) is recommended. Taste is important, as always eating bland food is boring and can leave you feeling like you want more.

Your bowel movements are also an important consideration. You should have regular bowel movements once or twice a day. They should be firm and occur without gas or cramping. If you experience cramps, it could mean that something you ate has caused some type of blockage or wind. Observing your stool can provide some clues to problems:

- Partially digested food or stools that are not brown may indicate that the food did not suit you or you may have eaten too quickly, without chewing adequately. Raw foods can be harsh to digest, and some people do better stir-frying or steaming their food.
- The presence of a lot of mucus may mean that the food is too cold or hot. White mucus indicates that something you have eaten is too cold. Brown or yellow mucus could indicate that you ate something too spicy or hot.
- Bubbles relate to excess stress or could be a sign of sugar intolerance (i.e. you may not be digesting sugar well).

Having constant watery saliva coming up into the mouth may indicate that the stomach has become very cold. It may also indicate that the yang energy in the digestive system is not working smoothly.

Craving sweet foods after a meal may indicate that your digestive system needs support. It may also indicate spleen weakness, calling for a good spleen-strengthening program to be implemented.

A sticky, bitter taste in the morning when you wake up or during the day may indicate heat in the stomach or gallbladder. A sticky taste could also come from dampness and a blockage in the mid-section. Paying attention to digestive imbalances or disturbances, and taking steps to rectify them, will help you adjust your weight.

CHAPTER THREE
Natural Ways to Enhance Beauty

In this section, you'll learn more about how to attain smoother, younger and more vibrant skin and hair, as well as achieve a healthy weight, using ancient Chinese wisdom about food and herbs.

We will also introduce some other time-honored traditional methods such as point acupressure, meridian massage and scraping, skin masks, tinctures, pastes, and herbal and foot baths.

1. Food and Herbs

Documentation about the many plants and foods that promote beauty and anti-aging can be traced back through Chinese history (fig. 12). Food is a part of everyday life, something to which we might not give much thought. However choosing the right foods and herbs is essential for health and beauty.

It is important to understand the different qualities and functions of the foods you consume to make appropriate choices for your individual constitution. You are unique and should therefore eat accordingly. The principles of choosing foods in relation to beauty are:

- Using flowers: Since ancient times, many beauty foods

have incorporated the flowers of certain plants. These can help the energy in your body to rise. They cause qi to flow smoothly, and blood circulation and meridians to open. They also help to nourish or regenerate the surface of the face and the upper portion of the body. Rose bud tea is a perfect example of this principle.

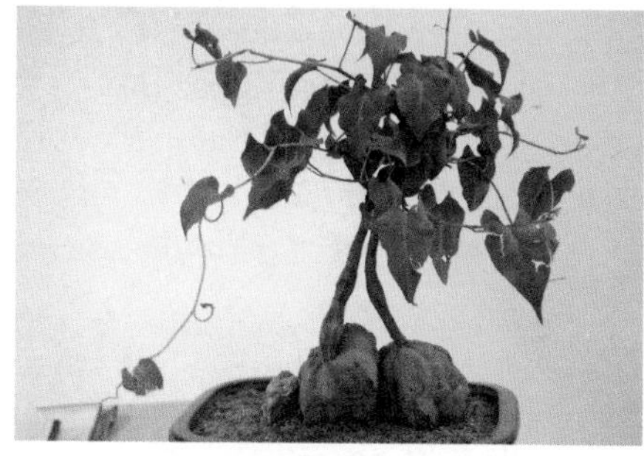

Fig. 12 Fo-ti root (Polygonum Multiflori, *he shou wu*) is a powerful anti-aging root.

- Strengthening qi and blood: Your beauty depends on the optimal function of every organ in your body, and each organ is fundamentally reliant upon qi and blood. Therefore foods and herbs that increase quantity or quality of qi and blood can enhance beauty. Examples include jujube, lychee, longan fruit and Chinese yam (*shan yao*).
- Promoting and regulating water metabolism: The body's surface is in direct contact with the outside world, so the surface of the skin can be more vulnerable to outside factors. This could affect the hydration of the skin and body or the amount of dampness coming into the body from the environment. It is important to make wise choices to suit your surroundings. For instance during a rainy damp season, it is prudent to consume foods and beverages that help eliminate excess water, like pearl barley or green tea. During dry seasons it is wise to choose foods and tonics that help to hydrate, like silver ear or wolfberries.
- Regulating the reproductive system: According to TCM

if you support the liver and kidney systems, they will manage the other organs in order to slow aging. Food and herbal remedies are often chosen for this purpose, and include Chinese angelica root (*dang gui*), wolfberry, motherwort (*yi mu cao*) and mugwort (*ai ye*).

2. Self-Massage

Massaging the acupoints of meridians and channels can unblock stagnation, improve blood and body fluid circulation, and increase metabolism of the face, eyes, hair, scalp and leg areas. We have included in following sections the massage techniques relevant to each specific beauty issue.

3. Natural Masks

Masks made from natural ingredients can be chosen according to skin type. Those with conditions relating to heat or with red burning skin may use cooling masks made with cucumber or the white parts of a watermelon.

Those who have cold conditions or very pale or puffy skin may use masks with hot towels that have a warming nature. One example is cinnamon and clove powder mixed with hot water and then applied with a hot towel compress, which can effectively reduce puffiness and bring rosiness to the skin.

A medical use gypsum facemask can be used to reduce pigmented skin or acne marks. Steam the face, massage the facial reflexology points, and apply the mask, which has been made with herbs and mineral water.

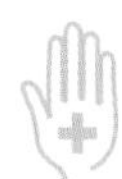

Essential Oils for Facial Massage

Facial massage is a good way to release toxins, relax face muscles and work on acupressure points.

Carrier oils such as jojoba, almond, hemp seed and coconut oil can be used, to which active essential oils may be added.

Rose, lavender and ylang ylang are all good essential oils to use for facial massage. You should use only one to three drops (added to a carrier oil) if you have sensitive skin (fig. 13).

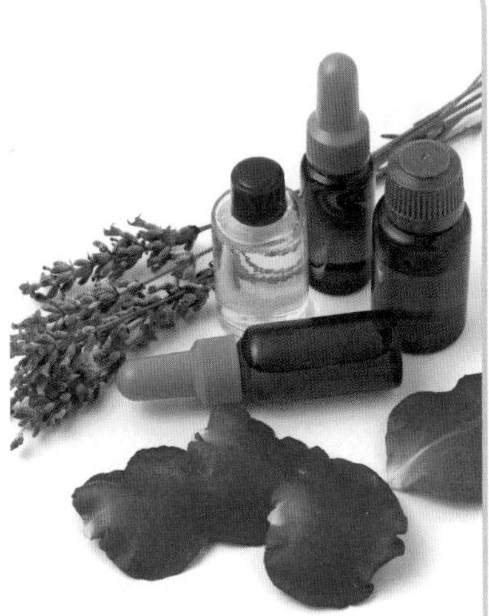

Fig. 13 Oils for facial massage

You can use 1 tsp of carrier oil with two to three drops of essential oil and one vitamin E capsule.

Please be aware that not all oils are suitable for all people. For instance those who are pregnant cannot use certain oils, while those with high blood pressure may also need to monitor which oils they use. You should do your own research according to your own situation.

Rosemary oil: Yang, warm, spicy and sweet, it goes to all five organ meridians. It is good for calming the mind and can be helpful in aiding digestion. It is great for dandruff and helps to combat poor hair growth. It also helps to open the glands, especially the reproductive glands.

Rose oil: Warm in nature, it goes to the liver and spleen. It helps to regulate the flow of energy and promote blood circulation, and it has a harmonizing effect on spleen qi and liver blood.

Lavender oil: Fairly neutral, it promotes relaxation of the skin and mind. It is a healing and anti-aging oil.

Clove oil: Great for the body, it helps stimulate sexual activity and can counteract low sex drive. It is warm and spicy, and helps to improve digestion and reduce nausea. It can tonify qi and goes to the meridians of the kidney, spleen, lung and stomach. It can warm the organs, especially reducing stomach coldness, and strengthens kidney yang.

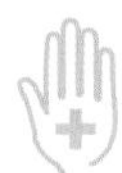

Hydrating and Nourishing Face Mask

This facial mask will leave your skin hydrated and reduce facial redness.
Ingredients: 25 g silver ear, 1 L water, 2 vitamin E capsules
Preparation:

1. Wash and soak the silver ear overnight.
2. Bring to a boil, then simmer for 45 minutes until it is soft and can easily be broken apart.
3. Strain mixture, preserving the liquid. For this mask you will only use the liquid. The rest of the silver ear can be mixed with yogurt or honey to nourish your inner organs.
4. Place the liquid into a small bowl and add two capsules of vitamin E. The texture should become like a gel, which is similar to aloe vera (*lu hui*).
5. Wait until it cools. If it is too runny then you have added too much water.
6. There are two application options. First, you may apply the gel directly to your face and leave on for 15 minutes. Reapply as often as needed during this time period as it might absorb into the skin quickly. The second option is to use a facemask. Using paper or silk, cut to the size of your face, creating holes for the eyes, nose and mouth. Soak the cloth in the gel, then place it on your face. This mask can be washed and reused.
7. Wash face after treatment and apply a nourishing cream.

4. Other Options

Pastes can be used by mixing dried herbs with a small amount of fluid for topical applications. Herbal baths, for the body or just the feet, can be created by adding ginger, mugwort or sulphur powder.

5. Top Ten Super Herbs for Beauty

In this section, you will learn about important characteristics of plants, according to TCM. This includes details about the properties, tastes, channels of entry, composition, pharmacology, culinary usage and medical applications of the ten most celebrated plants in Chinese medicine. These herbs are vital to maintaining inner health, and therefore, outer beauty.

Rose Bud 玫瑰

Scientific name and origin: Rose buds are flowers of Rosaceae, with the Latin name *Rosa rugosa* Thunb. Within China, they are native to the northern part; however they are now found all over China, sourced mostly from Zhejiang and Jiangsu provinces.

Properties and taste: Warm; sweet, bitter.

Channels of entry: Liver and spleen.

Composition and pharmacology: Rose buds contain rose oxide, a-naginatene, quercetin and cyanin. They increase microcirculation of the cardiovascular system, and have anti-viral and anti-oxidant effects.

Medical applications:

1.Regulating flow of qi: Rose buds can regulate the body's energy and qi movement. They ease symptoms of PMS, including breast tenderness and distention, as well as irregular menstruation.

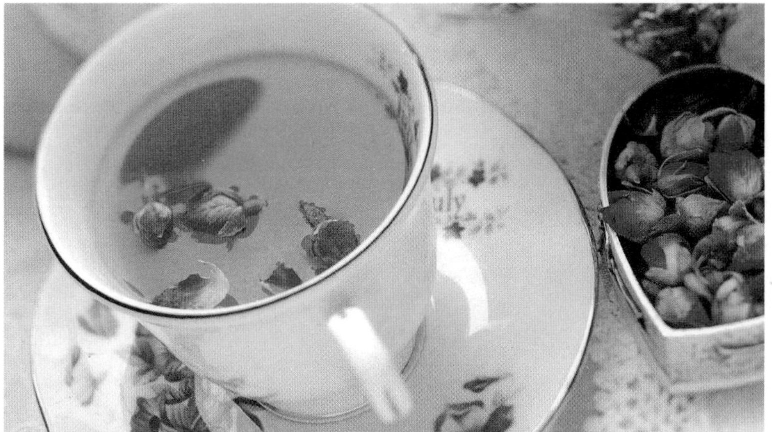

Fig. 14 A cup of tea using dried rose buds

Rose buds can help break up and dissolve crystallized breast tissue, which would otherwise grow into small lumps. To ease stomach pain and side pain (underneath the ribs), rose buds are often used.

2.Promoting circulation of blood: Rose buds are noted for improving blood circulation especially to the extremities and poorly oxygenated organs or tendons. They work to stabilize water content in blood while balancing the proportions of red and white blood cells, T-cells and platelets to improve overall blood function.

3.Unique harmonizing effects on both qi and blood: Rose bud is noted for its function on both qi and blood; therefore it is used to bring color back to the face and warm the hands, especially in cold weather. Likewise, tendonitis sufferers, women prone to excessive soreness when wearing high heels, or people who have recently suffered an injury or experience more than mild soreness should drink rose bud tea to enhance both qi and blood circulation to those areas.

How to eat:

When using dried rose buds in any of the below preparations, generally three to six buds are used.

1.Tea: Dried rose buds are commonly brewed into tea (fig. 14).

2.Desserts: Because of their sweet nature, rose buds can be incorporated into a variety of desserts. To enhance a dessert soup, first soak the dried rose buds allowing them to open up, and then select the best looking ones. Prepare a sweet soup of glutinous rice and sesame balls (which can be bought at Asian markets), adding the rose buds to the boiling water for more flavor and color. Eat the whole soup, including the buds, and drink the liquid. Rose buds (soaked and selected as described above) can also be used to decorate a cake or other dessert.

3.Flour: After grinding the rose buds into powder, the flour can be mixed with baking flour to produce cakes, muffins or sweet bread.

4.Wine: Alternatively the buds can be placed in wine, leaving them to infuse, then drinking.

5.Decoction: A decoction using dried rose buds will help symptoms of PMS.

6.Raw: If fresh rose buds are available, and the source is good, this is another option. However the concentration of medicinal properties is not as high in fresh buds, so 10 to 15 buds (3–10 g) should be eaten.

External use:

1.To counteract stagnation of qi and dissipate blood stasis, use 5 g of rose buds in water for a bath or to soak feet for 20 minutes.

2.High quality essential rose oil can be used to massage the face, back, shoulders and other areas on the body. Rose oil is warm and can tonify the liver and spleen. It helps to regulate the flow of energy, promote blood circulation, and harmonize spleen qi and liver blood.

3.Rose bud extract can be used to make a mask. To prepare the mask, simmer 200 g of rose buds in water until they become very soft. Then discard the rose buds and simmer the remaining liquid over a low heat for two hours until it has a paste-like consistency. This paste can be mixed with honey and applied to the face.

Contraindication: Rose buds essentially have no contraindications.

Safflower and Saffron Crocus 红花 番红花

Scientific name and origin: The Latin name of safflower is *Carthamus tinctorius*, of the family Asteraceae; saffron crocus belongs to the family Iridaceae, and its Latin name is *Crocus sativus* L. Its native regions are from southern Europe to Iran. Within China, safflower (*hong hua*) is commonly grown in Henan, Yunnan,

Sichuan, Zhejiang and Jiangsu, and is ready for harvesting in the summer. Saffron grown in Tibet and Europe becomes ready in the autumn.

Properties and taste: Warm; spicy (safflower). Neutral; slightly sweet (saffron crocus).

Channels of entry: Heart and liver.

Fig. 15 Dried safflower

Composition and pharmacology: Saffron crocus (*fan hong hua*) contains crocin and crocetin. It acts as a blood thinner, and increases uterine motion and low blood pressure. It has anti-cancer properties, and can improve memory and learning capacity.

Medical applications:

1.Strengthening the blood, promoting circulation: Both strengthen the blood, but safflower focuses more on circulation while saffron crocus is better at nourishing blood.Through their effect on blood, they can ease pain caused by blood stagnation, such as menstrual or post-partum pain, or lower abdominal pain. Both can address amenorrhea or delayed menstruation, as well as induce labor contractions.If post-partum discharge lasts beyond 15 days, safflower is prescribed to speed up and terminate the process.

2.Treating dry skin and swelling: For dry, scaly, flaky, purplish skin, safflower can help resupply blood to those areas. Safflower is also useful for acute injuries that are accompanied by swelling and bruises.

How to eat:

When using safflower, 6–9 g is the typical daily dosage, while for saffron crocus, 0.5–1 g is recommended.In the winter, when vessels have a tendency to close up, half a dosage is sufficient to revitalize blood circulation, especially to the brain.

1.Tea: Dried safflower can be brewed into tea (fig. 15).

2.Spice: Dried saffron crocus is used in cooking.

3.Decoction: Safflower can also be made into a decoction or soaked in wine, and then taken as a drink.

4.Granules: If granules are available, they can be used for tea, mixed into juice or sprinkled on top of salad.

External use:

1.Safflower oil: Widely available in Chinese pharmacies, it can be used to massage aches and pains.

2.Bath: Use 10 g of dry safflower to make an herbal bath or 3–5 g for a footbath. Soak for 20 minutes.

Contraindication:

1.Pregnant women must not eat safflower, except in the circumstances specified above.

2.Avoid if menstruation is heavy.

3.If you do not suffer from blood stagnation, there is no reason to take safflower as a medical supplement.

Lychee 荔枝

Scientific name and origin: Lychees are fruits of Sapindaceae (Soapberry family). Latin name: *Litchi chinensis* Sonn. The earliest record of lychees is from the Song dynasty (960–1279) in China. They mainly grow in the southeast, east and southwest provinces of China.

Properties and taste: Warm; sweet, acid.

Channels of entry: Liver, spleen.

Composition and pharmacology: Lychee contains glucose, proteins, vitamin C and lemon acid.

Medical applications:

1.Producing bodily fluid and nourishing blood: Lychee fruit quenches thirst, relieves cough, calms the mind, and relieves palpitations. It clears up acne, pustules, canker sores and

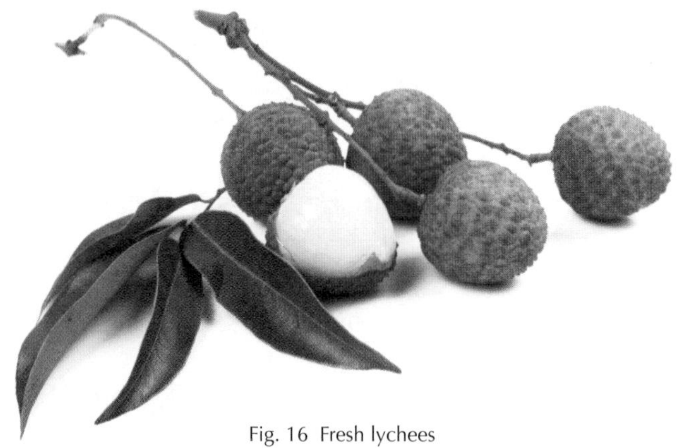

Fig. 16 Fresh lychees

mouth ulcers, and moisturizes face skin. Due to this function of nourishment, it is the "queen of fruits" for skin beauty.

2.Strengthening the spleen and liver: Through these qualities, lychees can treat stomach yin weakness marked by irritability, thirst, nausea and stomach ache. They also treat spleen deficiency, which otherwise could lead to lack of appetite or diarrhea.

3.Dispelling swelling and pain: Lychee seeds and plant bark can relieve pain and knots, tranquilize cough, and prevent and treat hernia.

How to eat:

1.Raw (fig. 16): Eating 50 g of fresh lychees can treat dry skin with wrinkles, thirst, toothache or soreness, and a swollen throat. For chronic diarrhea, eat fourteen lychees and ten jujubes for three days.

2.Dried fruit: For women with heavy and long menstruation, accompanied by fatigue and anemia, use 30 g dried lychee to make soup for five days. To improve qi and blood deficiency due to giving birth or senile weakness, use 20 g dried lychee and

100 g oats to make porridge for breakfast, and eat for a week.

3.Decoction: The following decoction can ease hernias with cold stomach, fullness, distention and abdominal pain. Boil 30–60 g of fresh lychee root to make a decoction. Add brown sugar to taste and drink for a course of five days.

4.Wine: Lychees are also made into fruit wine or potent liquor, which can warm the body and aid sleep. The following recipe can help impotence, premature ejaculation, mental and body fatigue, and weakness of the knees or lumbar area. Remove the skin of 500 g fresh lychees, soak in 500 ml high-percent alcohol wine for a week. Then drink 20 ml twice a day until finished.

Contraindication: If your body feels hot, dry and weak, with heartburn and constipation, or there is an accumulation of yellow phlegm, you should eat with caution.

Jujube (Chinese Date) 大枣

Scientific name and origin: Jujubes (*da zao*) are mature fruits of Rhamnaceae. Latin name: *Ziziphus jujuba* Mill. They mainly come from the Hebei, Henan and Shandong provinces of China.

Properties and taste: Neutral to warm; sweet.

Channels of entry: Spleen, stomach and heart.

Composition and pharmacology: Zizyphus saponin I, II and III, jujuboside B, stepharine, glucose and fructopyranose are all found in jujubes. Jujubes are a superb functional food, regulating body mechanisms, stopping coughing and reducing phlegm, and

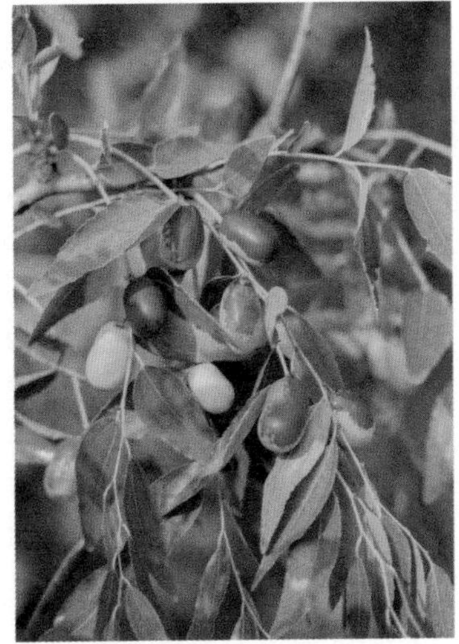

Fig. 17 Fresh jujubes

restraining nerve centers and calming the mind. Their anti-oxidants protect the liver; anti-cancer properties are also present.

Medical applications:

1.Strengthening the spleen and stomach: Jujubes can treat weak stomach and spleen, as evidenced by shortness of breath, tiredness, aversion to speaking, low appetite, sensations of fullness, distention of stomach and abdomen, and loose bowel movements.

2.Nourishing the blood to tranquilize the mind: Jujubes can ameliorate deficiencies of blood and spleen qi as manifested by insomnia, forgetfulness, palpitations of fear, and poor appetite. They are also useful for liver and heart blood deficiencies, with symptoms that may include irritability, hysteria, lassitude, mood swings, absent-mindedness, light sleeping, confusion, uncontrollable yawning, laughing or crying, thirst, constipation, and being easily affected by the environment.

3.Easing and reducing the toxicity of other herbs: Jujubes alleviate the side effects of medications. They can decrease the side effects of very strong herbs, and protect the spleen and stomach.

How to eat:

1.Decoction: Chop 10–30 g of dry jujubes, boil into a decoction for approximately 20 minutes. This can enrich the blood of the heart and strengthen spleen qi.

2.Stew: Wash and chop 250 g chicken and 30 jujubes into bite-sized pieces. Place into a heat-safe bowl along with 5 g ground ginger powder and 100 ml water. Steam for an hour, adding salt to flavor. This recipe can be good for men with sexual dysfunction or impotence caused by too much sex, often accompanied by dizziness and blurred vision, palpitation, shortness of breath and exhaustion.

3.Soup: Wash 60 g jujubes thoroughly; add 180–250 ml

of water, soak for 15 minutes, then boil for 20 minutes. Eat approximately 20 to 30 jujube and drink 50–80 ml of the soup daily for three days. This soup is good for weak and cold stomachs, stomach ache and poor appetite.

4.Fresh or dried (fig. 17): Eat five to ten jujubes daily, two to three hours before bed. If using fresh, be sure to wash thoroughly; cooked jujubes can also be used. This is good for insomnia.

5.Porridge: Cook 500 ml of water, 30 g jujubes, 120 g rice and 30 g dried longan fruit (skin and pit removed) together to make porridge. Eat one bowl, twice a day. This can nourish the heart, ease the mind, strengthen the spleen, and enrich blood. It is good for people with palpitations, insomnia, amnesia, anemia, spleen weakness with diarrhea, edema, spontaneous perspiration and night sweats, characteristics of both qi and blood deficiency.

6.Paste: Stew jujubes for about an hour. Remove the skin and pit, and pound into a paste adding sugar to taste. This can be used instead of butter or jam on toast or accompanying any other food.

Contraindication: Jujubes are not suitable for people with phlegm accumulation or poor appetite caused by indigestion.

Silver Ear (White Fungus or Tremella) 银耳

Scientific name and origin: Silver ear is a dry sporocarp of the Tremellaceae family. Latin name: *Tremella fuciformis* Berkeley. Silver ear is commonly grown in China's Sichuan, Fujian, Jiangsu, Zhejiang, Anhui and other nearby provinces.

Properties and taste: Neutral; sweet, bland.

Channels of entry: Lung, stomach and kidney.

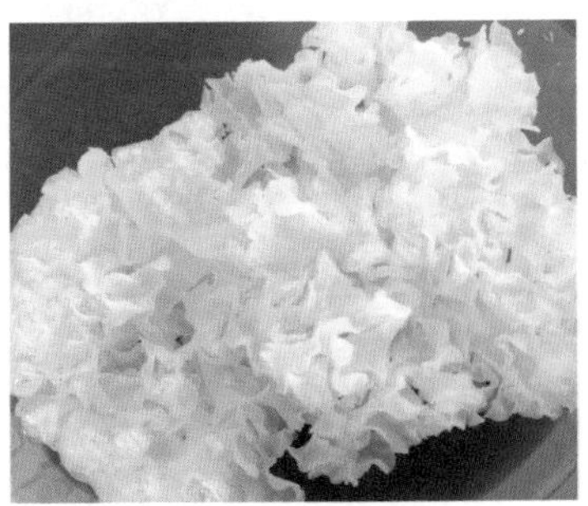

Fig. 18 Sweet dessert with silver ear

Composition and pharmacology: Silver ear mainly contains tremella polysaccharide, protein, fat, crude fiber, inorganic salt, vitamin B, enzymes and amino acids. It strengthens the immune system, aids protein synthesis and helps the body generate new blood. Silver ear is believed to counter aging and fatigue as well as the effects of radiation. It can reduce lipids in the blood, moderate blood sugar, prevent tumors and ulcers, and act as an anti-inflammatory.

Medical applications:

1.Nourishing yin and promoting body fluid: Silver ear helps weak constitutions after illness, shortness of breath and lack of energy. Those who have low blood pressure or have hearing difficulties (often caused by changes in air pressure on airplanes), should use silver ear with lily bulb.

2.Moistening the lung and strengthening the stomach: Silver ear can strengthen lung qi, indicated by weak, chronic or dry cough, and thick discolored mucus, often accompanied by chest pain or tightness. It is noted for its ability to nourish fluids in the digestive tract, reduce dry mouth and constipation, quench thirst, and reduce both stomach and mouth ulcers.

How to eat?

1.Porridge: Silver ear is popular in rice porridge, such as Eight Treasures Porridge.

2.Dessert (fig. 18): It can be incorporated into sweet desserts; silver ear steamed with papaya is a tasty and popular dessert.

3.Decoction: Silver ear decocted with astragalus root can raise the white blood cell count.

External use: Thoroughly cook 5 g of silver ear. Separate the juice and solids. Apply the juice on the face or other dry skin area.

Contraindication: People with a cough (particularly a productive cough with thick yellow or green phlegm), liquid sputum or aversion to cold should use with caution.

Poria 茯苓

Scientific name and origin: Poria is the sclerotium of the polyporaceae family. Latin name: *Poria cocos* (Schw.) Wolf. Poria comes from a dried fungus. China's main supplies come from Yunnan, Anhui and Hubei provinces.

Properties and taste: Neutral; sweet and bland.

Fig. 19 Poria

Channels of entry: Heart, spleen, lung and kidney.

Composition and pharmacology: Poria can stimulate the regeneration of tissue and mucus. It can reduce blood pressure and open the vessels close to the heart. It eases upset stomach by reducing acidity, and also reduces toxins.

Medical applications:

1.As a diuretic to expel dampness and treat water retention: This herb is useful for those who either have normal or scant urine, a bloated abdominal region caused by water retention, or a feeling of heaviness.

2.Strengthening and harmonizing the spleen and stomach: It has been used to treat spleen and stomach weakness especially where there are conditions of poor appetite, soft stool or diarrhea, and mental or physical fatigue.

3.Calm the heart and mind: Poria can be used to help spleen and heart disharmony and weakness. Conditions such as heart palpitation, insomnia, forgetfulness, lightheadedness and lack of appetite may be treated using this herb.

How to eat:

1.Herbal tea: Add 45 g poria (fig. 19), 45 g dried tangerine skin, 15 g licorice root and 15 g ginger. Grind them into a powder, then each day use 5 g in boiling water and drink. Take for three days.

2.Soup: Add 10 g poria and 10 g wolfberries to 150 ml water, and cook to make a special thick soup.

3.Steamed: Take 120 g of poria (skin removed), chop into bite size pieces, then steam. Use as a snack whenever you feel hungry. This is useful for those who have a lot of vaginal discharge or frequent urine.

4.Edible paper: In China poria is often used to make wafer-thin paper to wrap around dried fruit. Use 100 g poria powder, 100 g Chinese yam root powder and 200 g starch or glutinous rice powder. Add warm water and mix until you have a thick paste. Then cook pancakes (wafer-thin) using very low heat on an iron plate or non-stick pan. This recipe can also be used to make paper for spring rolls, or pancakes for Beijing duck. It will strengthen the spleen and help those with a poor appetite, and is beneficial for children with bed wetting issues. It can also help with weight reduction.

External use:

1.Face mask: Use 20 g poria powder and mix with honey. Apply to the face before going to bed and wash off in the morning. This mask will nourish facial skin and reduce pigmentation.

2.Tincture: Use 10 g poria, 20 g psoraleal (Psoralea corylifolia L, *bu gu zhi*), and 20 g eclipta (*mo han lian*). Put all the herbs in 200 ml of 75% alcohol. Soak for one week. Then strain, reserving the liquid. Apply the herbal liquid to bald patches once or twice a day to help hair regrowth.

Contraindication: When taking poria internally, do not consume any vinegar or foods with vinegar on the same day.

Wolfberry 枸杞子

Scientific name and origin: Wolfberry is a mature fruit of Solanaceae. Latin name: *Lycium barbarum* L. It is found in Ningxia, Gansu and Xinjiang provinces in China.

Properties and taste: Neutral; sweet.

Channels of entry: Liver, kidney, lung.

Composition and pharmacology: Wolfberry contains betaine, wolfberry LBP-I, polysaccharide acid, multi-vitamins and minerals. Research shows that wolfberry can help boost and regulate the immune system. Also wolfberry helps with iron deficiency and anemia, and can increase white blood cell count. It has anti-cancer properties, reduces high cholesterol, high blood sugar and high blood pressure. Overall it protects the function of the liver and has anti-aging properties.

Medical applications:

1.Strengthening the liver and kidney, nourishing essence: Wolfberry helps nourish and enrich the yin and essence of the liver and kidney. It can help with lower back and knee pain, as well as tinnitus, insomnia, nightmares, spontaneous emission and early onset of aging.

2.Promoting blood products and healthy eyes: It can be used to improve eyesight (near- and far-sightedness) as well as dizziness.

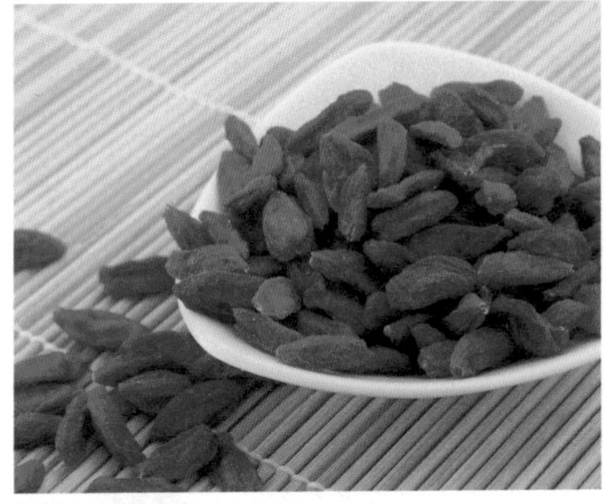

Fig. 20 Wolfberries

3.Controlling diabetes symptoms: Clinically, wolfberry has also been used to control symptoms such as increased thirst and blood sugar swings.

How to eat:

1.Steam: Steam the wolfberries, then stir fry with mixed vegetables. They may also be used as a garnish and sprinkled on top of all types of dishes and desserts.

2.Snack (fig. 20): Let the berry soften in your mouth and chew it slowly.

3.Soup: Mix water and wolfberries, using one cup of water for every 10–15 berries. Simmer for five minutes, and drink the soup and eat the berries.

4.Tea: Mix three bulbs of chrysanthemum flowers with ten wolfberries in a cup. Pour in hot water, put a lid on and let brew for five minutes. Drink while warm. If preferred the wolfberries can be ground into powder and then mixed with hot water.

5.Porridge: Mix 15 g wolfberries, 100 g glutinous rice or 50 g oats, and 250 ml water. Cook for 20 to 30 minutes, and add a bit of honey or jujubes if you want a sweeter flavor.

6.Jelly or pudding: Take 200 g wolfberries, 200 g longan fruit and 2000 ml water, bring to a boil and then let simmer for two hours. Discard the extra liquid and continue to cook on a low heat until all the ingredients have a jelly- or pudding-like consistency. Consume two teaspoons twice daily, morning and night (the above quantity is for about three weeks). This jelly is particularly beneficial for nourishing the blood and yin-yang, calming the mind and sharpening memory, and strengthening tendons and bones.

7.Wine: Wolfberries mixed with alcohol will make wolfberry wine.

8.Decoction: You can boil the berries with eucommia bark for a decoction to treat lumbago.

Contraindication: People who suffer from diarrhea or are easily prone to developing mucus in the throat and nose should use wolfberry with caution.

Chinese Angelica Root 当归

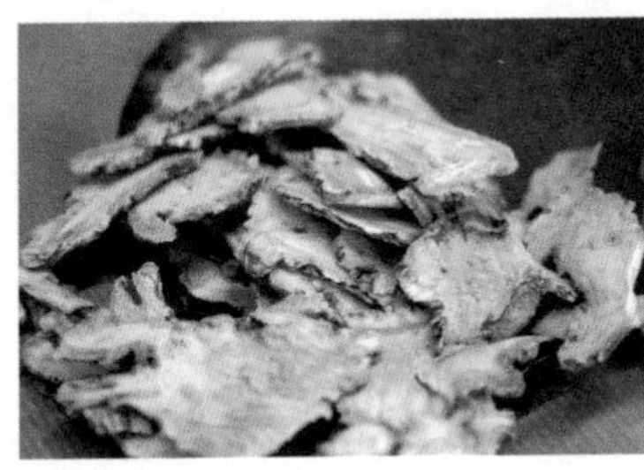
Fig. 21 Chinese angelica root

Scientific name and origin: Chinese angelica is a root of Umbelliferae. Latin name: *Aaugellica sinensis* (Oliv) Diels. It is mainly produced in southeast Min County (Qinzhou) of Gansu province in China.

Properties and taste: Warm; sweet, pungent, bitter.

Channels of entry: Liver, heart and spleen.

Composition and pharmacology: Chinese angelica root has volatile oil (ligustilide) and water solubility (ferulic acid), as well as polysaccharide, amino acid, vitamins and natural elements. It can strengthen both specific and nonspecific immunity, and improve hemopoiesis. Furthermore it protects the liver and is an anti-oxidant. It also acts against radiation, regulates heart rate, increases the flow of the coronary artery, reduces the oxygen consumption of the myocardium, dilates vessels, brings down peripheral resistance, prevents thrombus, and breaks down blood fat. It can be applied as a two-way regulator of uterine contraction, or to prevent inflammation, relieve asthma, induce analgesia, and in clinical tests, has been shown to fight germs and tumors.

Medical applications:

1.Tonifying the blood and promoting blood flow: Chinese angelica root acts to tonify the blood, and it can also regulate blood circulation. It is effective in treating symptoms such as pale face, dizziness, vertigo, palpitation, poor memory, insomnia, fatigue and lassitude due to blood deficiency or the deficiency of both qi and blood. Furthermore it is effective in treating numbness, tremors, stiff neck, and muscle weakness due to deficiency and stagnation of blood.

2.Regulating menstruation and alleviating pain: It can not only be used in promoting blood flow to regulate menstruation but also in tonifying the blood. It is one of the key herbs used in obstetrics and gynecology, and is widely applied in cases of irregular menses, dysmenorrhea, amenorrhea, postpartum abdominalgia and uterine bleeding. However it can be used to treat pains in all parts of the body, such as headache, abdominal pain, numbness with stiffness and spasm of limbs, and even for pain associated with injury as well as ulcers and sores induced by infection.

3.Loosening the bowels to relieve constipation: The nature of Chinese angelica root is to nourish and moisten; therefore it can be used in treating dryness of the intestine due to blood deficiency, especially in a weakened older person and or someone with blood deficiency due to childbirth. Typical manifestations are weak, difficult excretion with dry stool, pale face, palpitation, shortness of breath, insomnia, memory problems and pale tongue with white fur.

How to eat:

1.Decoction (fig. 21): Use a slice of chinese angelica root (5–15 g) together with other herbs. Put the herbs into an earthenware pot with 500 ml of water to stew for 45 minutes, pouring off and reserving the liquid. Add another portion of water and cook again. Then add this to the first batch of liquid, and stir well. Drink half in the morning and half in the evening for menstrual discomfort.

2.Medicated wine: Ancient records mention using chninese angelica root for medicated wine in treating arthralgia (joint pain).

3.Soup: Make a soup with ginger and mutton.

4.Powder: Chinese Angelica root can be ground into powder for pills.

External use: Chinese angelica root can be applied as a facial mask. You can buy angelica cream from an herbal pharmacy. Apply to skin once or twice a week to help rough skin or pigmentation.

Contraindication: The nature of Chinese angelica root is warm, so those who have yin deficiency in the stomach, lung yin deficiency with heat, kidney weakness with damp-heat, and liver-yang excess with phlegm-fire should use with great caution. It should also be used with care in cases of excess damp-heat, or damp-heat blocking the digestive system accompanied by loose stool.

Mugwort (Argy Wormwood Leaf) 艾叶

Scientific name and origin: Mugwort comes from the leaves of the Asteraceae family. Latin name: *Folium Artemisiae* argyi. China's main supplies come from Anhui and Shandong provinces.

Properties and taste: Warm; spicy and bitter.

Channels of entry: Liver, spleen and kidney.

Composition and pharmacology: Mugwort contains volatile oil, flavonoid, triterpenes and many minerals. It can fight against pathogenic microorganisms and serve as an anticoagulation. It stops bleeding and cough, and removes phlegm. It is an anti-inflammatory, anti-cancer and antimutagenesis agent that can boost immunity.

Medical applications:

1.Warm the uterus and stop bleeding: It is especially effective in treating bleeding caused by spleen yang deficiency (when the body feels cold,

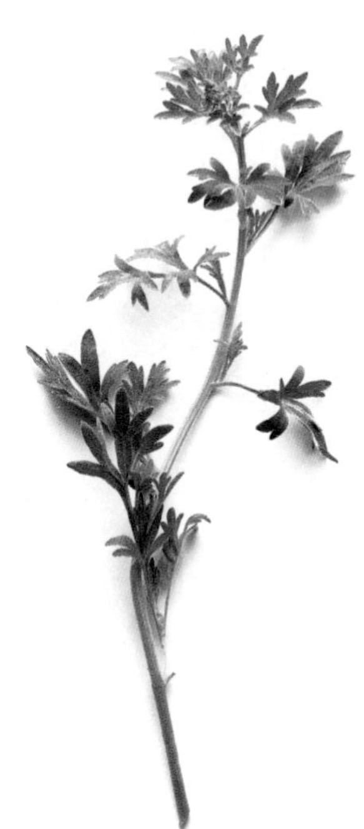

Fig. 22 Mugwort

blood is pink and watery, and bleeding lasts longer than usual).

3.Regulating qi movement and blood circulation: It helps people who feel heavy and cold in the lower back and abdominal area.

4.Expelling cold and dampness: It is particularly good for treating cold abdominal pain and diarrhea.

How to eat:

1.Juice with fresh leaves (fig. 22): Wash 100 g of fresh mugwort leaves thoroughly. Put all the leaves in a juicer, add 30 ml water, and blend for 20 seconds. Finish the juice within 20 minutes. Add three pieces of dry ginger as an option. This juice can treat coldness in the hands and stomach coldness.

2.Decoction: Use 3–10 g of the dry herb to make a decoction. Wash thoroughly and chop into large pieces. Put in a pot with cold water. Bring to a boil, and after one minute reduce heat to lowest setting, simmering for 20 minutes. Strain the decoction, preserving the liquid. Add with boiling water into cup, and drink warm. You can make a 3-day supply at one time to treat long-term bleeding during menstruation with a weak and cold pattern.

3.Pill or powder: There are many famous ready-made powders and pills using mugwort, such as *Ai Fu Tiao Jing Wan*. Take 3 g of pills, twice a day, to treat the cold type of painful periods.

External use:

1.Moxibustion: You can buy moxa sticks and use them to treat cold, painful or stiff areas. For example to treat cold pain in the stomach, light the moxa until glows red. Place it 1.5 cm away from the Liangmen point for two minutes. The skin at that point will get pink and feel warm.

2.Decoction for skin: You may also use dried mugwort leaves (from a local pharmacy) to make a decoction. Add 60 g of cooked mugwort to 300 ml water. Bring it to a boil and then simmer for 15 minutes. This herbal liquid can be used for external wash, treating itchy skin. Apply the decoction locally to skin fungus or wart viruses. You can also use this decoction for a foot bath to treat cold feet.

Contraindication: Those with a hot constitution or yin deficiency (night sweating, five palm heat, constant thirst) should use the moxa option with caution. Moxa should not be used when bleeding excessively (for instance as a result of an accident).

Motherwort (Leonurus Cardiaca) 益母草

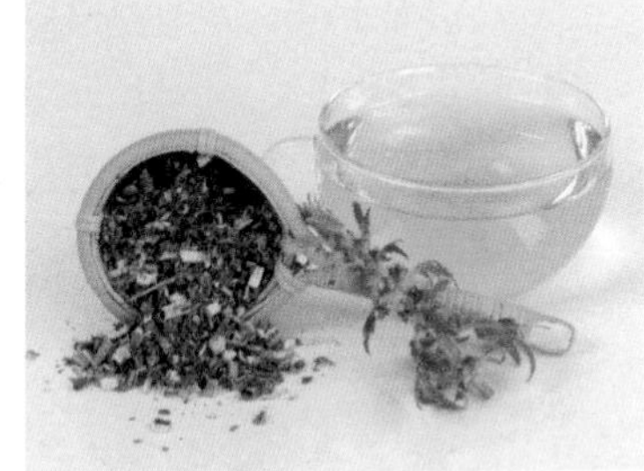

Fig. 23 Motherwort and motherwort tea

Scientific name and origin: Motherwort is the leaf of the Labiatae family. Latin name: *Herba Leonuri*. China's main supplies come from Henan, Anhui, Sichuan, Jiangsu and Zhejiang provinces.

Properties and taste: Slight cold; spicy and bitter.

Channels of entry: Liver, kidney and pericardium.

Composition and pharmacology: Used for centuries as a tonic for the female reproductive system, this plant contains bitters, terpene, tannins and alkaloids. It is a commonly used herb for regulating the menstrual cycle and easing pain, and for stopping bleeding. It stimulates activity of the uterus muscle, regulating range, frequency and tension. It fights platelet aggregation, and has anti-thrombogenesis and anti-myocardial ischemia properties. It also protects the kidney and improves cell immunity.

Medical applications:

1.Regulating blood circulation and menstruation: Motherwort is often used to treat irregular periods, amenorrhea and bleeding during pregnancy. It can also treat those who experience a feeling of collapse in the lower back and abdomen. It has been used to remedy difficult labor, dull complexion, dry and rough skin, and abdominal pain due to blood stagnation.

2.As a diuretic to remove swelling: It treats dysuria, edema and acute injury with muscle swelling and pain.

3.Cooling heat and expelling toxins: It can reduce carbuncle, heat rash and boils.

How to eat:

1.Ground form: You can buy motherwort plaster (*yimucao gao*) or motherwort powder (*yimucao keli*) from a TCM pharmacy to treat irregular periods. It is also available in pill form.

2.Decoction (fig. 23): Take 30 g of motherwort and 30 g of purslane, and cook as a decoction. Drink for nine days. This recipe is for long and heavy menstruation, and vaginal blood discharge after child delivery.

External use:

1.Soaking liquid: Grind fresh motherwort with a mortar and pestle, and then soak a cotton ball in the herbal liquid. Apply cotton ball to painful and swollen areas of the breast to treat mastitis.

2.Decoction for wash: Add 60 g of dry motherwort to 300 ml of water. Bring to a boil, then simmer for 15 minutes to make an herbal liquid for external wash. You can use it to treat acne and related scarring.

Contraindication: Those with yin and blood deficiency, heavy menstruation (weak and cold constitutions), and conditions where the pupils of the eyes are constantly dilated should avoid taking motherwort.

CHAPTER FOUR

Self-Assessing Your Five Organ Systems and Body Constitution

This chapter contains two parts. The first is a questionnaire for each of the five organ systems. The other is for assessing your body constitution.

1. Assessing Your Five Organ Systems

Completing the following questionnaires will help you discover which organ systems need priority care. The category that has the most "yes" responses is the organ system you should pay attention to first. If you are fortunate enough to have answered "yes" three or fewer times in any one category, then follow the star rating system discussed in Chapter Two.

After you have strengthened or regulated the weak organ system for at least two months, take the quiz again to reassess.

Questions Relating to the Heart System

1) Do you have trouble sleeping at night?

□ yes □ no

2) Do you have heart palpitations?

□ yes □ no

3) Do you have sweaty hands?
☐ yes ☐ no

4) Are you forgetful?
☐ yes ☐ no

5) Do you have circulatory problems?
☐ yes ☐ no

6) Do you feel nervous often?
☐ yes ☐ no

7) Do you frequently get ulcers on your tongue?
☐ yes ☐ no

8) Is your sleep often disturbed by nightmares or stressful dreams?
☐ yes ☐ no

9) Do you have an irregular heartbeat?
☐ yes ☐ no

10) Do often feel unhappy?
☐ yes ☐ no

Questions Relating to the Liver System

1) Do you regularly experience premenstrual syndrome (PMS) symptoms?
☐ yes ☐ no

2) Are your nails brittle or cracked?
☐ yes ☐ no

3) Do you often feel moody and cranky?
☐ yes ☐ no

4) Do you have a high stress lifestyle?
☐ yes ☐ no

5) Do your eyes tear frequently?
☐ yes ☐ no

6) Do you often feel irritable or restless?
☐ yes ☐ no

7) Do you regularly experience blurred vision, or dry, red and/or swollen eyes?

☐ yes ☐ no

8) Do you have tendon problems?

☐ yes ☐ no

9) Do you often get migraine headaches?

☐ yes ☐ no

10) Do you often feeling uncomfortable in your rib area (on both sides) and/or the top of your head and temples?

☐ yes ☐ no

Questions Relating to the Spleen System

1) Do you have severe food allergies or do you get food poisoning more than twice a year?

☐ yes ☐ no

2) Do you have sensitivities to certain foods?

☐ yes ☐ no

3) Do you often bloated after eating?

☐ yes ☐ no

4) Do you have heartburn?

☐ yes ☐ no

5) Do you often have diarrhea?

☐ yes ☐ no

6) Do you frequently have bad breath?

☐ yes ☐ no

7) Do you often have an upset stomach or nausea?

☐ yes ☐ no

8) Do you bruise easily?

☐ yes ☐ no

9) Do you dislike the wet season or damp weather?

☐ yes ☐ no

10) Do you have muscle problems (weakness, tightness, stiffness, knots, muscle tears)

☐ yes ☐ no

Questions Relating to the Lung System

1) Are you particularly susceptible to colds or flu?
   ☐ yes ☐ no
2) Do you have frequent coughs or asthma?
   ☐ yes ☐ no
3) Do you often experience shortness of breath?
   ☐ yes ☐ no
4) Do you have sinus problems?
   ☐ yes ☐ no
5) Do feel sad often?
   ☐ yes ☐ no
6) Do you often have a sore throat, throat tickle, mucus or the need to regularly clear your throat?
   ☐ yes ☐ no
7) Do you have hay fever?
   ☐ yes ☐ no
8) Do you often have skin issues?
   ☐ yes ☐ no
9) Do you smoke?
   ☐ yes ☐ no
10) Do you have constipation?
   ☐ yes ☐ no

Questions Relating to the Kidney System

1) Do your ears ring?
   ☐ yes ☐ no
2) Do you experience pain in your back, knees or heels?
   ☐ yes ☐ no
3) Do you have infertility or low sperm count?
   ☐ yes ☐ no
4) Do you have low sexual interest?
   ☐ yes ☐ no
5) Do you have frequent urination?

□ yes □ no

6) Do you have hair loss?

□ yes □ no

7) Do your bones or teeth break easily?

□ yes □ no

8) Are you experiencing menopausal symptoms?

□ yes □ no

9) Do you find it difficult to completely empty your bladder?

□ yes □ no

10) Do you have fear or panic attacks?

□ yes □ no

2. Assessing Your Body Constitution

A person must understand his or her own constitution in order to take the right steps to find good health. The assessments below will help you learn more about your own constitution in order to choose foods and herbs specifically suited to your individual needs.

Questions Relating to Temperature: Neutral, Cold, Hot or Mixed Constitution

1) Are you sensitive to the cold or heat?

□ normal (1) □ sensitive to cold (2)

□ sensitive to heat (3)

2) What do you prefer to drink?

□ depends on season (1) □ warm/hot drinks (2)

□ cold drinks (3)

3) Do you sweat a lot?

□ normal (1) □ less than average (2)

□ more than average (3)

4) How do you classify your thirst?

□ normal (1) □ not often thirsty (2) □ often thirsty (3)

5) How is your complexion?
□ shining and rosy (1) □ pale and puffy (2)
□ flushed (3)

6) How is your tongue coating when you get up in the morning?
□ thin white fur (1) □ thick white fur (2)
□ thick yellow fur (3)

7) What is your pulse (beats per minute)?
□ from 60 to 80 (1) □ less than 60 (2) □ over 80 (3)

8) Do you like tea or coffee?
□ up to two cups of coffee or tea everyday (1)
□ three or more cups of tea everyday (2)
□ three or more cups of coffee everyday (3)

9) What kind of food do you prefer?
□ depends on season (1)
□ a light taste or raw food (2)
□ spicy or strongly flavored (3)

Assessment (fig. 24):
Neutral: 6 or more responses of (1)
Cold: 6 or more of (2)
Hot: 6 of more of (3)
Mixed: if fewer than 6 of any one response

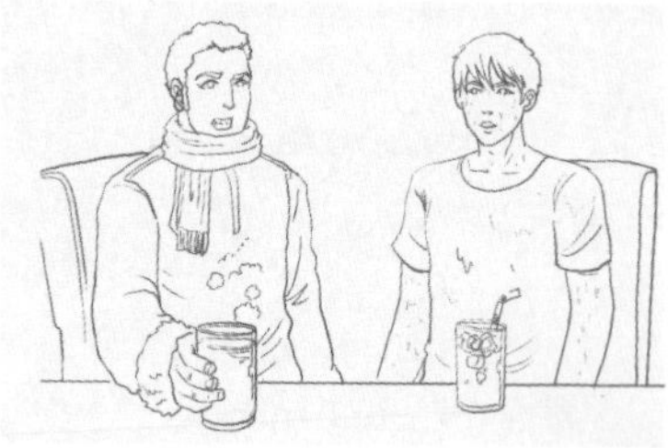

Fig. 24 Cold or hot

Questions Relating to Humidity: Neutral, Damp, Dry or Mixed Constitution

1) What is your tongue like?
□ normal size with a thin white coating (1)
□ large with a thick or wet coating (2)
□ small with a thin or dry coating (3)

2) What kind of taste do you usually have in your mouth?
□ normal (1) □ sticky and sweet (2) □ dry (3)

3) What is your skin condition?
   □ normal or mixed (1) □ oily (2) □ dry or cracking (3)
4) How would you characterize your excretion? (Discharge from eyes, ears and skin; for women, includes monthly period)
   □ comfortable amount (1) □ quite a lot (2)
   □ scant or absent (3)
5) Do you smoke or drink alcohol?
   □ occasionally (1) □ frequently (2)
   □ refrain from both (3)
6) What is your tolerance for dairy products?
   □ average (1) □ less than average (2)
   □ more than average (3)
7) How do you feel in general?
   □ happy and relaxed (1)
   □ heavy, sleepy; fullness of chest and stomach (2)
   □ irritable, anxious; dry lips and throat (3)
8) How would you characterize your bowel movements and urine output?
   □ normal (1) □ loose stool or turbid urine (2)
   □ dry stool, constipation or scanty urine (3)
9) How would you describe your build?
   □ average (1)
   □ heavy build (2)
   □ slim (3)

Assessment (fig. 25):
Neutral: 6 or more responses of (1)
Damp: 6 or more of (2)
Dry: 6 or more of (3)
Mixed: if fewer than 6 of any one response

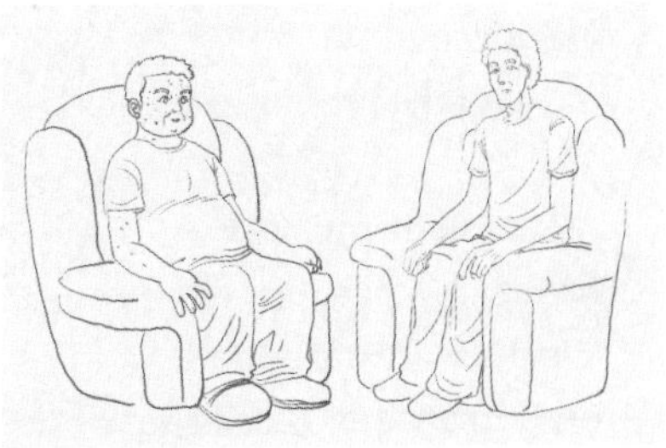

Fig. 25 Damp or dry

Questions Regarding Your Response to Adversity: Neutral, Weak, Overly Strong or Mixed Constitution

1) Do you feel energetic?
   □ average (1) □ more than average (2)
   □ less than average (3)
2) What is your tongue like when you get up in the morning?
   □ pink body and thin fur (1)
   □ dark or purple body and thick fur (2)
   □ pale or deeper red body and no fur (3)
3) What kind of food you prefer?
   □ mixed, with more vegetables and less meat (1)
   □ mostly meat (2) □ vegetarian (3)
4) How often is your elimination?
   □ normal (1) □ infrequent (2) □ too frequent (3)
5) How often do you get a cold every year?
   □ once or a few times (1) □ never (2) □ often (3)
6) How often do you get excited?
   □ normal (1) □ frequently (2) □ seldom (3)
7) How do your muscles feel?
   □ normal (1) □ tight and sore (2) □ soft and weak (3)
8) How quickly do you feel shortness of breath when hiking?
   □ 15 minutes to half an hour (1)
   □ more than half an hour (2) □ after a few minutes (3)
9) How does your head often feel?
   □ normal (1) □ pressure or sharp headache (2)
   □ lightheaded or dizziness (3)

Assessment (fig. 26):
Neutral: 6 or more responses of (1)
Weak: 6 or more of (3)
Overly Strong: 6 or more of (2)
Mixed: if fewer than 6 of any one response

Fig. 26 Weak or overly strong

In completing the above self-assessment, we encounter some pairs of concepts: cold or hot, damp or dry, overly strong or weak. All these feelings, when within a certain range, are normal for us to feel. We should feel cold in winter and hot in summer. However, if we always feel cold, even in spring, or feel cold too often, then we should seek the underlying reason and try to remedy it.

The approach toward damp and dry is similar; both are necessary and normal within boundaries. Dampness nourishes our inside and moistens the surface of skin while dryness limits the growth of mold. However, too much damp makes skin oily and develop acne. In turn, too much dryness brings wrinkles and cracking. Therefore we should stay in neutral as long as we can.

Now that you have assessed your constitution, we can use that information in choosing the right foods and herbs to help you achieve and maintain balance.

Let's take damp, dry and neutral constitutions as an example. If you have a result of a neutral type, it means you are quite balanced. In order to keep this state, it is best to eat a broad range of foods and be sure to drink water according to the climate and your level of perspiration. However, if you have a damp constitution, this means there is too much humidity inside of you. You need to add specific foods to your diet (such as pearl barley, azuki beans, corn) to reduce dampness and bring yourself back to balance. A dry type, on the other hand, would have different requirements for a healthy diet. In this case, foods such as lily bulb, Chinese wolfberry, honey or lemon can nourish and moisten the body.

PART TWO

ORGAN SYSTEM ANALYSIS

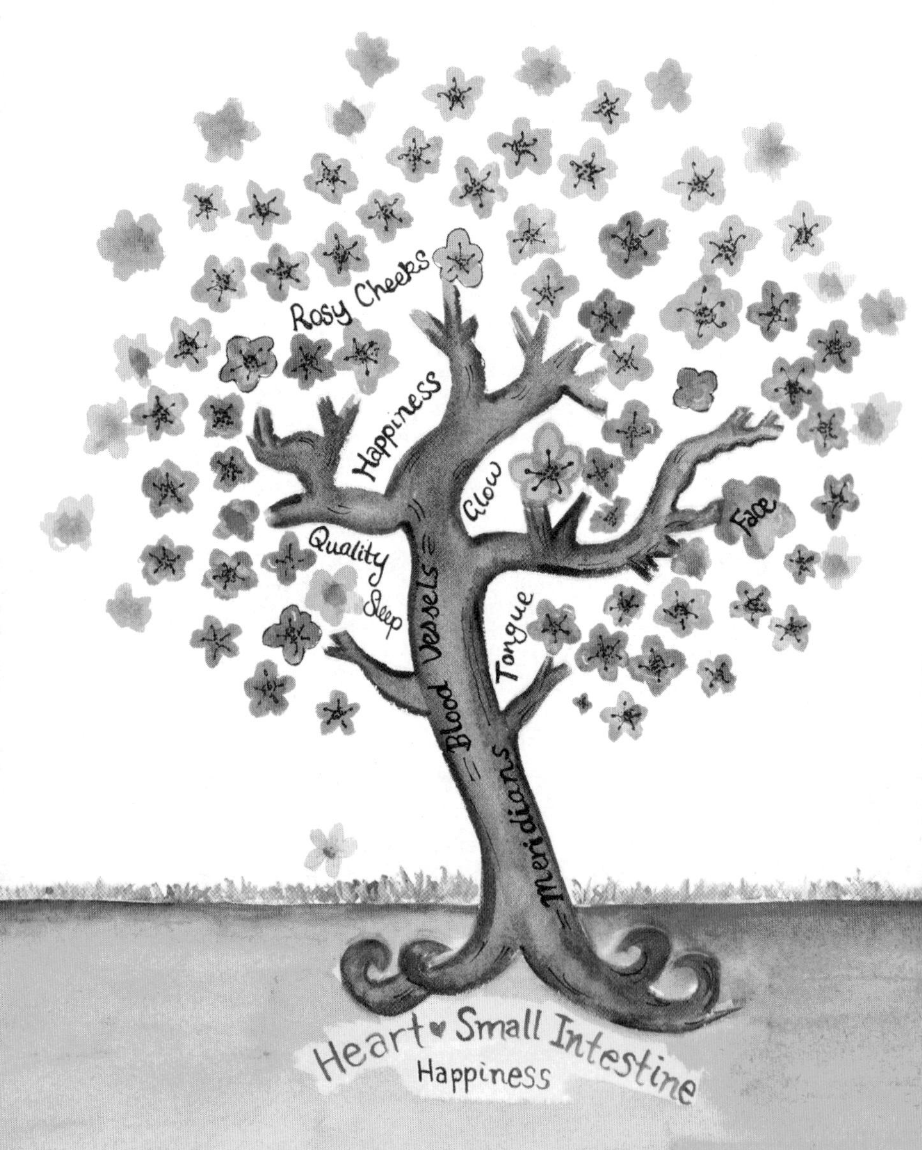

Rosy Cheeks
Happiness
Glow
Face
Quality Sleep
Blood Vessels
Tongue
Meridians
Heart Small Intestine
Happiness

CHAPTER FIVE

The Heart System

Roots

- *Zang*-organ: heart
- *Fu*-organ: small intestine
- Mental heart: includs mind and spirit, and emotions of happiness and joy

Trunk and Branches

- Blood vessels: all the body's blood vessels
- Meridians: Shaoyin Heart Meridian of Hand, Taiyang Small Intestine Meridian of Hand

Leaves

- Pink tongue
- Rosy cheeks
- Emotional sweat

Fruits

- Quality sleep
- Emotion of happiness (also part of the "roots" system)

Flowers

- Beautiful glowing complexion on face

Left Fig. 27 The heart system tree

1. Basic Facts about the Heart System

As we learned previously, in traditional Chinese medicine the heart system includes the heart, small intestine, blood vessels, meridians and tongue. When we discuss the heart, we are referring to both the "physical heart" and the "mental heart".

The "physical heart" plays a significant role in governing blood and controlling the blood vessels, and thus regulates the entire body's physical functions. It is involved with circulating blood and qi, and providing nourishment to every cell.

The "mental heart" refers to its function of dominating mental and spiritual activities. In many Chinese medical texts, the heart is considered to be the "house" of the spirit (*shen*) and the "emperor" of the body. Since the way a person views life can have a profound effect on health, the role of the "emperor" is critical. It helps to govern various emotions as well as your nervous system and brain.

Effective heart function produces a peaceful mind and facilitates the movement of nourishing blood throughout the body. It is vital for longevity and beauty.

From a TCM diagnostic point of view, the physical heart and mental heart are complementary. A relaxed mental state and smooth blood circulation will carry nutrients to nourish all the cells, and these nourished cells create a glowing complexion on your face. So let's take a deeper look into the heart system and its functions.

2. Function of the Physical Heart: Blood and Blood Circulation

The heart controls the blood in two ways. First, the transformation of nutritive qi and body fluid into blood takes place in the heart. Second, the heart is responsible for the circulation of blood (fig. 28).

Blood circulation is important for maintaining healthy cells that produce a vibrant body. Healthy circulation is dependent

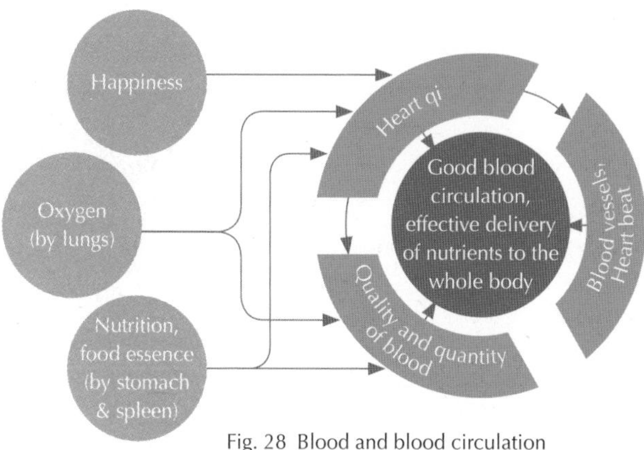

Fig. 28 Blood and blood circulation

upon heart qi, the quality and quantity of blood, and an absence of blockages in the blood vessels. When these factors are all present, they ensure endless and smooth blood circulation.

According to TCM, heart qi is produced from oxygen (created as a result of a healthy lung system) and nutrition (formed from strong stomach and spleen systems). Heart qi is vital, helping to produce blood, and serving as the driving force for the movement of the heart muscles. It also contributes to the elasticity of the arteries, veins and capillaries. It is responsible for regulating a normal heartbeat and ensuring the blood vessels are moving in the same rhythm.

Food essence, especially nutritive qi and body fluid (managed by a well-functioning stomach and spleen), kidney essence, and normal function of the lung and heart, ensure the quantity and quality of blood.

Blood is circulated in the blood vessels effectively when heart qi is functioning well. Optimal quantity and quality of blood, as well as its good circulation, ensures the effective delivery of nutrients to the whole body. When heart qi moves smoothly the blood also flows effortlessly. If heart qi begins to move too slowly the blood will accumulate "stagnation".

Assessing the Physical Heart through External Examination

There are many physical signs that communicate whether or not your heart is working effectively. A TCM doctor might examine the color of your complexion and your tongue's appearance, measure your pulse, and perform a physical examination of your chest to determine whether the heart system is functioning optimally. There are further physical characteristics that speak volumes about heart function, as categorized below:

- Good heart function: Rosy cheeks with hydrated, glowing skin. Pink tongue with free movement. Firm and regular rhythm of the pulse and a comfortable feeling in the chest.
- Heart qi deficiency: A pale face with dull skin tone, and a swollen, pale colored tongue. A weak pulse and in more extreme cases chest palpitations with feelings of weakness. Heart qi deficiency may also present as dull aches or tingling in the arms.
- Stagnation in the blood or blocked blood vessels: Bluish-purple and gloomy face. Purple dots on the tongue or a purple tongue body. Chest palpitations with a feeling of fullness. Chest pain or pressure with pins and needles. An irregular and astringent pulse.

3. Function of the Mental Heart: Mental Activities and Emotional State

According to TCM theory, the heart governs the mind, which refers to clarity of consciousness and the strength of mental and emotional faculties. In Western physiology, these are considered functions of the brain, but in TCM they are linked directly to the organs, with the heart system considered particularly important.

In the narrow sense, *shen* is a collective term for cognition, consciousness and mental activities such as memory and quality of sleep. However in the broad sense, *shen* also manifests in

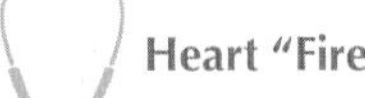

Heart "Fire"

Physical symptoms of heart fire include:

- Palpitations
- Thirst
- Mental restlessness
- Feeling agitated
- Insomnia
- Ulcers or red sores
- Redness on the tip of the tongue

These symptoms can occur when the heart doesn't adapt to the environment in summer. TCM would describe this condition as the heart being invaded by heat. It can also occur when a person has many mental or spiritual concerns. If one doesn't find a way to rebalance, relax and adapt to stress quickly, internal "fire" or "heat" can develop.

The symptoms above are a result of the body attempting to expel excess heart fire. The excess heat can also show up as chronic bladder infections, which can be brought on by stress, a hot body system, or hot/humid seasons.

physical appearance and mannerisms, linked with all the organs. For instance, your confidence level, how you dress and speak, your ability to maintain eye contact, and the way you interact with the world around you are all a reflection of your *shen*.

The specific emotion linked to the heart in TCM is happiness or overexcitement. Being happy helps to harmonize your heart qi, and can influence sleep and the distribution of nourishment to the tissues and cells. In times of extreme emotions, your body will send blood and nutrients to the organs, so your skin and external features might not receive optimum nourishment. Happiness is therefore important to ensure great heart function and a beautiful complexion.

Assessing the Mental Heart through External Examination

A TCM doctor will question you to examine your mental activities, such as state of happiness, consciousness, memory and sleeping patterns, and can categorize the results as follows:

- Good heart function: Normal mental activity, balanced emotional life, clarity of consciousness, good memory and sound sleep.
- Heart blood and qi deficiency: Unhappy, depressed, poor memory, insomnia and sleep that is disturbed by stressful dreams.

4. Meridians of the Heart System

The Shaoyin Heart Meridian of Hand originates from the heart and connects internally with the small intestine. The superficial channel appears under the armpit and runs down the inner side of the arm down toward the tip of the smallest finger (fig. 29).

The Taiyang Small Intestine Meridian of Hand begins at the tip of the smallest finger and then runs up along the outside of the arm. It makes its way to the back of the shoulder, up the neck and across the cheek, and finishes near the corner of the eye. Internally it connects with the heart and small intestine (fig. 30).

The pericardium is intimately connected with the heart and small intestine, since it is attached to the heart from the perspective of structure and meridian. It is also linked with the *san jiao*, which separates the body trunk into upper, middle and lower portions. Both these organs have meridians that also travel down the arm; these are the Jueyin Pericardium (fig. 31) and Shaoyang *San Jiao* Meridians of Hand (fig. 32). Together with the two meridians mentioned in the previous paragraph, these meridians are vital for the healthy function of the arms. The skin, tendons, lymph circulation, blood vessels and muscles all rely on these four meridians to carry qi and blood to nourish the arms.

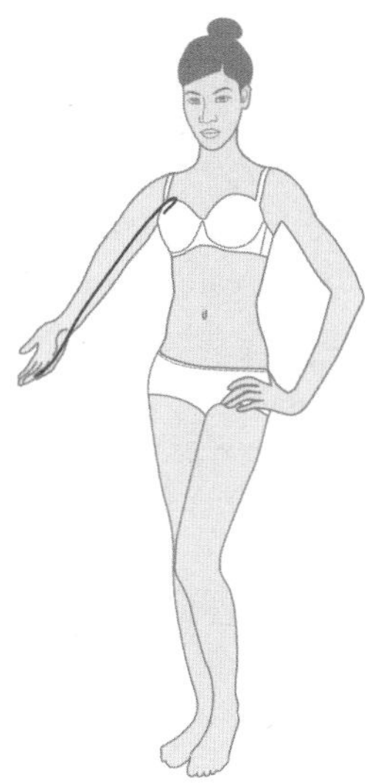

Fig. 29 Shaoyin Heart Meridian of Hand

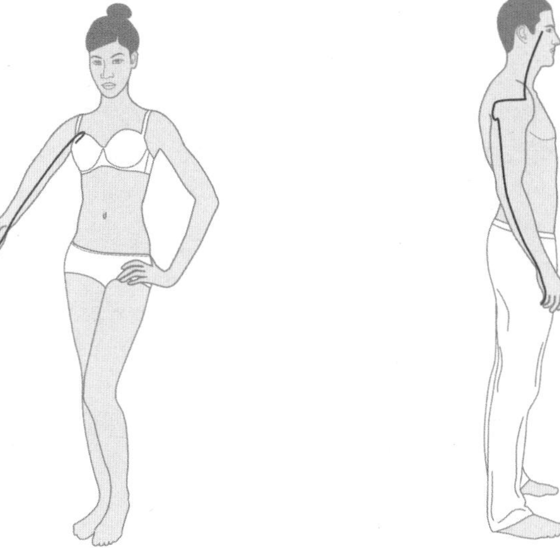

Fig. 30 Taiyang Small Intestine Meridian of Hand

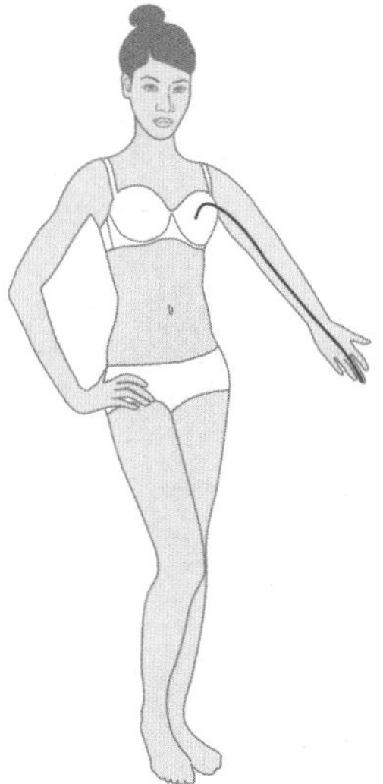

Fig. 31 Jueyin Pericardium Meridian of Hand

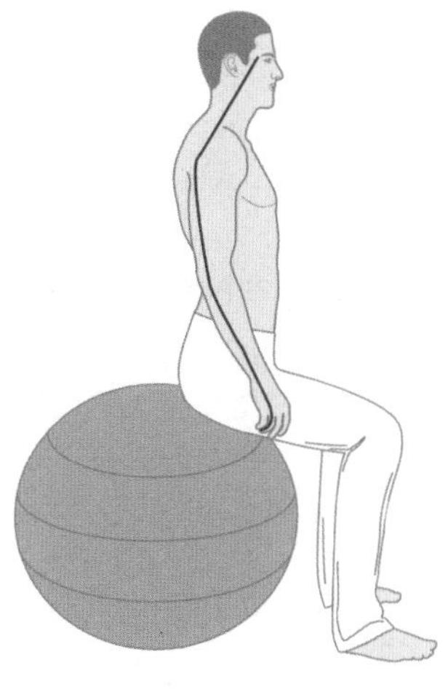

Fig. 32 Shaoyang *San Jiao* Meridian of Hand

5. Heart System and Beauty

A strong heart system will help the body maintain healthy blood and blood vessels. The blood vessels should be elastic with the ability to shrink or enlarge according to the outside environment and other bodily factors. So in addition to a lovely complexion, excellent circulation and motor coordination are dependent upon the heart system.

In TCM, the emotion of happiness and the ability to govern all emotions effectively play a part in keeping the heart system healthy. Thus there is a relation of mutual dependence between the function of controlling blood and that of regulating the mind.

Face: Flower of the Heart

When talking about beauty, the first thought is usually facial beauty. There are a few aspects to facial beauty: cheeks, eyes, hair and skin. Aside from congenital factors, beauty is reliant on health. Since we will explore these aspects in depth later, here we will focus mainly on the complexion relating to three points: color, moisture and shine. A glowing, hydrated and rosy complexion is highly valued (fig. 33).

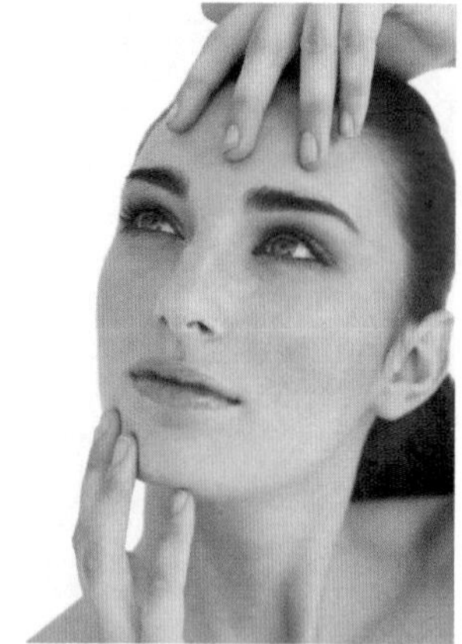

Fig. 33 A glowing, hydrated, and rosy face complexice is highly valued.

- Color: Although somewhat dependent on skin color, in most cases a beautiful face should have pinkness in hue. Dullness paleness, or a yellow and purple color will reduce attractiveness. Pink beneath the surface of the skin may indicate sufficient quantity of blood and smooth blood circulation through the blood vessels.
- Moisture: A lovely face also

should be well hydrated, with soft, smooth skin. Dryness, wrinkles, puffiness or sagging will detract from beauty. So the heart plays a role in creating the ideal texture for your skin through the effective delivery of nourishment. A healthy heart system can help prevent unsightly veins.

- Shine: An attractive face must be glowing, showing positive emotion. Unnaturally dark or dim skin will make people wonder about your health. A glowing complexion also depends on the quality of sleep, which the heart plays a role in regulating.

Pulse: Measure of the Heart

A strong, calm, regular heartbeat is important for heart health. In most cases, normal heart function includes a heart rate of 60 to 80 beats per minute; the heart rhythm should be regular, consistent and even. The intensity of your heart rate should suit your age, fitness level and lifestyle.

The frequency, rhythm and intensity of the pulse are all examined to determine normal heart function. Someone with very poor heart qi may find it difficult to do daily tasks, such as carrying heavy items, and may feel fatigued all the time. He or she may have a pale complexion, irregular pulse, palpitations, dizziness and the inability to deal with stress.

Tongue: Sprout of the Heart

In Chinese medicine, the tongue is the "sprout" of the heart. It means that the tongue is the cross station of blood vessels. It also builds a bridge between the meridians of the Conception Vessel and Governing Vessel when practicing *qi gong*. TCM doctors regularly observe the tongue to give them a picture of what is going on internally. When a TCM doctor looks at your tongue they are looking at several things:

- Tongue body: The sides and foundation of the tongue. The

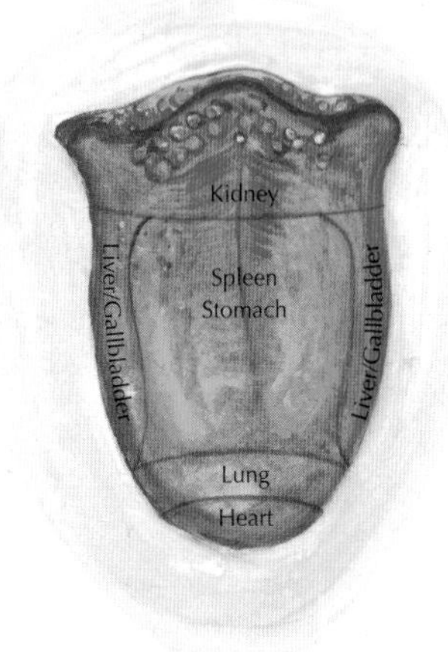

Fig. 34 Tongue and its five related organs

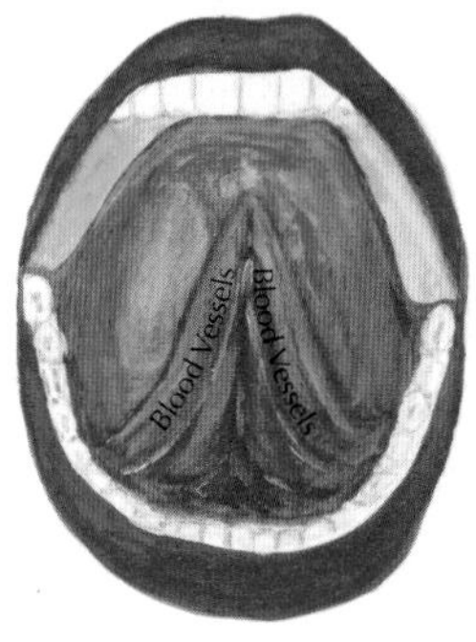

Fig. 35 Underneath the tongue and its related organs

appearance of the tongue should be pink, soft and hydrated.

- Tongue function: This includes smooth speech and sensitive taste. The body of the tongue should be coordinated and move freely, helping expression through speech.
- Tongue coating: The surface of the tongue.
- Specific regions: There are certain sections that correspond to each organ. The tip of the tongue is related to the heart (fig. 34).
- Blood vessels: The blood vessels underneath the tongue indicate if blood is flowing well or stagnated. They should be light blue, not too thick or too purple. A dark purple color in this region might indicate there is blood stagnation (fig. 35).

If there is heart qi deficiency (yang deficiency), the tongue will become pale and large in size, because it will hold more water. If heart blood deficiency (yin deficiency) is present, the tongue will be deep red and become smaller due to lack of body fluids. Ulcers and red spots or sores on the tongue can be indicative of heart fire, especially when accompanied by a very red tongue.

Happiness: Emotion of the Heart

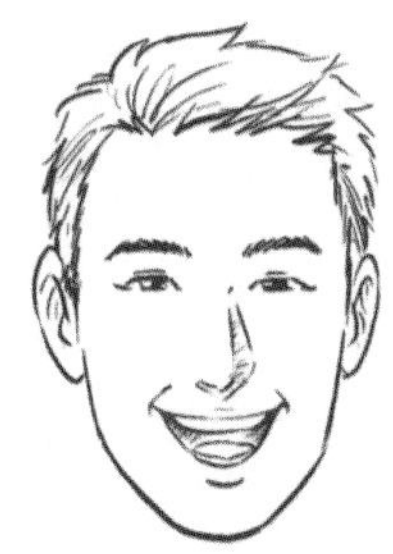

Fig. 36 Happiness is a positive emotion.

As we have seen, happiness relates to the heart system and the element of fire. Happiness is considered to be a positive yang emotion that tends to make energy flow upward and outward.

For instance when you are happy, the corners of your mouth and eyes move in an upward and outward direction, while internally the energy in your muscles is also travelling upward (fig. 36). Happiness relaxes qi and blood as well as helping to balance emotions. An opening effect occurs, including the opening of your mind, heart and blood vessels. Your body has more oxygen when you are happy.

On the other hand, overexcitement can actually make one act abnormally or feel unbalanced. This emotion can raise blood pressure and make the heart beat too fast, which of course in not healthy over the long term. When you have extreme emotions, your body will send blood and nutrients to your organs, depriving your exterior, including your skin. This is why happiness is important to ensure great heart function and a beautiful complexion.

6. Beauty Problems and Enhancements

Now we will discuss how to strengthen the heart system to maintain rosy cheeks, sound sleep, smooth circulation and good water metabolism in the heart and small intestine meridians.

Sometimes the heart system gets out of balance. Symptoms include blood disorders, irregular or rapid pulse, sweaty palms, nervous tension, inability to sleep, extreme redness in the face, and cold hands and feet. Some arm swelling and pain in the heart meridians might also be a sign that your heart system needs attention.

Achieving Beautiful Rosy Cheeks

Rosy cheeks are a sign of good health. However sometimes imbalances will cause excess redness, purple, paleness and/or dryness to occur.

1) Imbalance: Redness (with or without Spider Veins)

Too much redness in the face can be a frustrating beauty concern. There may or may not be spider veins present. According to Chinese medicine, facial redness can be caused by an excessive hot constitution or yin weakness. Other causative factors can include superficial capillaries, a hyper sympathetic nervous system, and sensitivities or allergies.

First of all, you need to assess the cause. Do you have the symptoms of excess or weakness?

Symbols of Excess Body Heat	Symbols of Weakness of Yin
Feeling hot in the whole body, not just in the face	Red cheeks with hot flushes, or five palm heat
Thirsty, prefer cold drinks	Dry mouth and throat, night sweats, weight loss
Red tongue with yellow coating	Empty feeling in chest. Red tongue with no coating
Yellow urine	Scanty urine

A. Caused by Excess Body Heat

If your condition is caused by excess heat, you must balance your body. On a short-term basis, you can cool the body externally by using a face cloth with ice water or moving into a cooler spot. However for more lasting results, you must turn your attention internally to cool the excess heat. Avoid spicy food and red meat, and increase your vegetable and fruit intake, being sure to select those with a cooling nature.

Prolonged redness in the face can encourage the formation of spider veins due to the fact that the capillaries are constantly expanded. Prevention is easier than a cure.

The following foods are recommended:

- Watermelon, as a fruit or juice.
- Lotus plumule tea with a slice of lemon and honey.
- Mung bean and mung bean sprouts, which are detoxifying as well as cooling.

Mung Bean Soup

Ingredients: 50 g mung beans, 450 ml water

Preparation:

1. Wash mung beans thoroughly.
2. Soak overnight or for at least a half hour.
3. Bring water to boil, then add pre-soaked mung beans to boiling water. Stir briefly.
4. Bring to boil again, simmer on low heat for about a half hour. Turn the heat off, leaving covered, and let the soup sit for five minutes.

Some people prefer to just drink the soup and not eat the beans. If this is your preference, 20 minutes cooking time should suffice.

Contraindication:

1. For someone with a cold stomach it is better not eat too much mung bean soup, although once or twice during summer should not cause excess coldness.
2. For cold constitutions, it is better to avoid having mung soup in winter. Instead hawthorn berries, which are warming to the body, will have similar detoxifying effects. Hawthorn berries also help with food poisoning and indigestion.

B. Caused by Weakness of Yin

For those who have a red face due to weakness, sensitivity and deficiency, rather than body heat, a different course of action should be taken. It is important to remove the food or environmental irritant and then to tonify the body fluids.

The following foods are recommended:

- Silver ear is an effective remedy for tonifying body fluids. It strengthens the immune system and is believed to

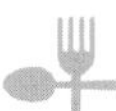

Mung Bean Sprouts

You can make your own mung bean sprouts. Mung beans are an excellent source of protein and take very little time to sprout; they will be ready to eat within two to three days. You can eat them once they have sprouted little tails (fig. 37).

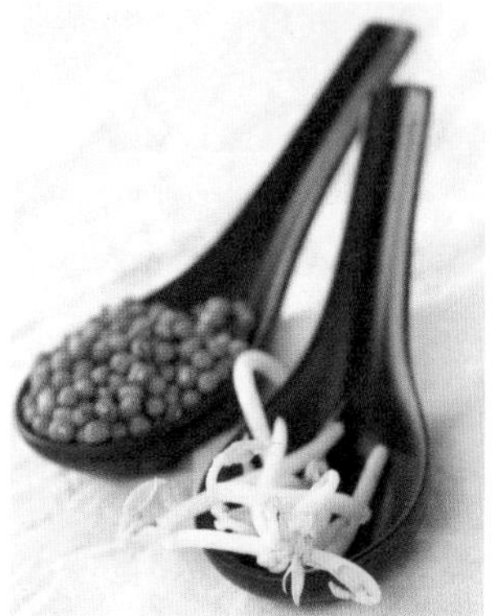

Fig. 37 Mung bean and mung bean sprouts

Tools: A clean bowl (it is recommended to sterilize it with hot water) and a cover (such as cheesecloth, paper towel or perforated lid)

Ingredients: two tablespoon mung beans; purified, filtered or spring water

Preparation:

1. Rinse the mung beans and put them in a bowl. Add water to a level about 3 cm above the beans, and leave to soak overnight.
2. On the next morning, drain the beans and put them back in the bowl. Cover with a cheesecloth or other material, and put in a dark cupboard. They need air, so don't use a tight lid.
3. Rinse and drain the sprouts. Usually only once a day is necessary but if they seem dry, a second rinsing and draining is helpful. Use caution however; if they are too wet, they can get moldy.
4. Once they are ready to eat, store the sprouts in the fridge. Continue to rinse every few days.

If you get mold or your sprouts don't turn out for one reason or another, just try again. You'll quickly develop a sense for when to rinse and drain them.

How to eat:

1. Raw: This method preserves many enzymes and antioxidants.
2. Fried: Quickly stir-fry for two to five minutes depending on whether you like them crisp or soft.
3. Soup: Add mung bean sprouts three minutes before you finish cooking noodles or any other kind of soup.

Contraindication: Compared with mung beans, the sprouts are not as cold in nature, so they are better tolerated by those with a cold constitution.

counteract aging and fatigue. It aids protein synthesis and helps the body generate new blood. Silver ear reduces lipids in the blood, moderates blood sugar, prevents ulcers, and acts as an anti-inflammatory. Furthermore it is thought to counteract the effects of radiation and prevent tumors. Silver ear can be used in a facial mask to treat redness and leave your skin hydrated.

- Beet (beetroot) is good for strengthening the heart meridian. It is neutral in temperature and sweet in taste. Beet contains phytonutrient biochanin-A, folate, betacyanin, vitamin C and beta-carotene. It can help lower blood pressure and reduce risk of heart disease. Therefore beet can be eaten to remove facial redness that is caused by high blood pressure in the early stages of heart dysfunction.
- Apple is effective for tonifying the body fluid of the heart. It is cool in temperature and sweet in taste. It prevents summer-heat from disrupting heart function, and treats facial redness, irritability and thirst.

2) Imbalance: Purple Spider Veins (with Facial Redness or Paleness)

Purple spider veins usually indicate deep-rooted constitutional blood stagnation. This can be caused by either a cold or hot condition, or a lack of body fluids.

When there is a cold condition in the body, blood can stagnate because the vessels shrink due to the cold body environment. This can leave blood trapped, leading to purple veins (usually on a pale face).

A hot constitution can also lead to spider veins. When someone has a chronically hot body condition, the liquid in the blood is consumed quickly, leaving a slow, sticky blood flow. Consequently circulation slows down, leading to stagnation. These spider veins will initially be red and then turn purple once stagnation has fully set in.

If the purple veins have been caused by stagnation from a cold constitution, then foods that warm the body can be used. If the condition is caused by a hot constitution, cooling foods or teas might help improve the fluidity of the blood. This will prevent the fluids from being used up too quickly, which will help improve circulation and remove stagnation.

The following foods are recommended:

- Grapes can regulate blood circulation, and are good for both cold and hot conditions. Purple grapes have stronger anti-stagnation properties. Either eat 100 g of grapes or blend them into a juice, including the skin and seeds.
- Red wine, in a small quantity (approximately 20 ml) is appropriate for both cold and hot conditions. Be sure not to consume too much if you have a hot condition.
- Hawthorn berries, both fresh and dry, are an effective tonic. They are also beneficial for liver, spleen and stomach function. Do not consume too much if you have a hot condition.
- Eggplants are useful for regulating blood stagnation caused by heat. They help to cool the blood and can alleviate some joint pain and rashes caused by heat. They can be steamed or stir-fried.

Contraindication:

1.It is important to note that having a lot of ice, or very cold beverages or food, is not recommended, as this is too extreme. The goal is to encourage subtle differences over a longer period of time, rather than suddenly introducing a lot of cold into the body. Regardless of whether the purple veins are caused by heat or cold, it is appropriate to regulate blood circulation of the heart.

2.If you suffer from spider veins it is important not to frequently engage in treatments such as chemical or fruit acid peels, steroids, microdermabrasion or scrubs. These can thin the skin over time and make veins more apparent for susceptible individuals.

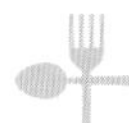

Hawthorn Berry Jam

Ingredients: 300 g fresh hawthorn berries (fig. 38), 300 g brown sugar (reduce to 150–200 g if desired), 150 ml water, half of a fresh lemon

Preparation Method One:

1. Wash the hawthorn berries thoroughly.
2. Add the water to a pot (avoid using iron), bringing it to a boil. Then add the hawthorn berries. After the water starts to boil again, simmer on a low heat for 20–30 minutes.
3. When the berries become very soft, use a wooden spoon to mash them. Allow the mixture to cool. Then drain through double-gauze to separate the seeds and jam liquid.
4. Bring jam liquid to a boil. Mix it with sugar slowly, in three steps: First add 100 g and stir well. After 20 minutes add another 100 g. Wait another 20 minutes, then add the remaining 100 g.
5. Add juice from the lemon, and stir thoroughly until a jelly consistency is attained. Store in an airtight container.
6. Use two teaspoons of this jam on top of pancakes or rice.

Preparation Method Two (if you do not mind the skin of the berry):

1. Wash the hawthorn berries thoroughly. Use clean scissors to remove the seeds.
2. Combine the berries and water in a blender for 60 seconds.
3. Pour into a stainless steel pan. Stir on a high heat, then simmer on low until the excess liquid has steamed off and there is a jelly consistency.
4. Add sugar and lemon juice, then mix well. Cool the jelly and put it into an airtight container.
5. Use two teaspoons of jelly as a filling for spring rolls or sweet dumplings.

Note: The final product from each of these recipes will last for 14 days in the refrigerator.

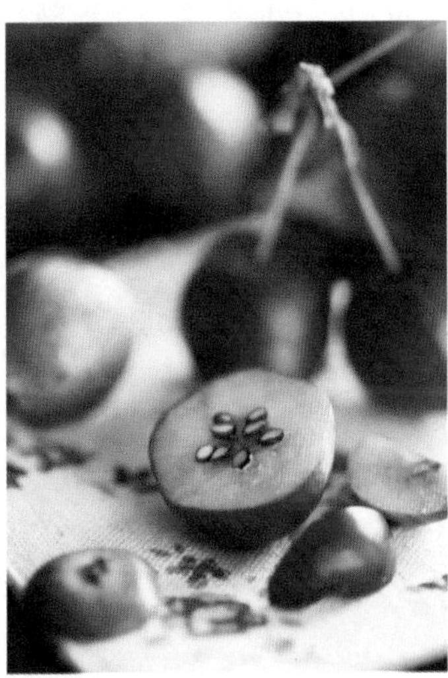

Fig. 38 Fresh hawthorn berries

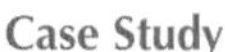

Case Study

Symptoms: Mrs. Wang, 49 years old, complained of facial skin redness, combined with expansion of the capillaries. Some areas of the face showed purple dots. She also experienced palpitation, chest pressure, and hot flushes in the afternoon and night. Her tongue showed a red tip and light yellow coating.

Treatment: To cool heart blood and nourish body fluid, herbal treatments combined with mint tea and lifestyle changes were implemented for a month. Her facial redness was reduced significantly.

Analysis: This condition, commonly known as "couperose skin", is caused by enlarged micro blood vessels. It can damage the facial or body skin. Although it can be in part hereditary, it can also be a sign of circulatory problems. The main reason for facial couperose skin is when the heart meridian accumulates heat, disturbing blood circulation. Clinically it affects women more.

3) Imbalance: Pale Face

Facial paleness is generally caused by a blood deficiency of the heart system. If you have such a blood deficiency, you might also feel light headed, weak and lacking in energy. Please keep in mind that when discussing "blood deficiency" here, we are referring to the TCM concept, which is defined by lack in blood quantity and poorly functioning blood. A sallow complexion, reduced memory, palpitation, insomnia and a pale tongue may be evident.

The following foods are recommended:

- Rose buds have a unique harmonizing effect on both qi and blood. They can be used to bring color back into the face and to warm the hands, especially in cold weather. Create a tea with 3 g of rose buds. You can also add 5 g of rose buds to your bath or in a basin of hot water for a footbath. Soak in the rose bud water for at least 20 minutes. Tendonitis sufferers, those who have recently had an injury, and those who experience body aches or pains can drink rose bud tea to enhance both qi and blood circulation to the affected areas.

Jujube Jelly

Ingredients: 250 g dried jujubes, 500 ml water, 25 g brown rice syrup or malt sugar, half of a fresh lemon

Preparation:

1. Wash the jujubes thoroughly, removing the seeds using clean scissors.
2. Soak jujubes in water for 30 minutes.
3. Blend the soaked jujubes with water for 60 seconds.
4. Take the liquid out of the blender and put into a stainless steel pan. Stir on a high heat, then simmer until the excess liquid has steamed off and a jelly consistency is attained.
5. Add sugar and lemon juice, mixing well. Cool the jelly and put into an airtight container to store in the refrigerator. The finished product will last 14 days.
6. You can use 15 ml each time, mixing it with water or eating it with bread.

Note: You can also use the jujubes for soup. Follow the same procedure (except you do not need to add the sweetener) and cook for 30 minutes. You can then drink the soup, and if you like, eat the jujubes as well.

- Jujubes help to tonify the blood and produce rosy cheeks with a glowing complexion. They can also help to produce shiny hair, good circulation to the lips and tongue, and an overall radiance. Consuming jujubes can reduce disturbed sleep with vivid stressful dreams.

Smooth Circulation

Strong heart qi, sufficient quantity of blood, and good function of the blood vessels are three essential components for blood circulation, which are all linked to heart. Problems with circulation can stem from several causes, which have different manifestations.

1) Imbalance: Cold Limbs

Some people only have cold hands and feet during the winter; others suffer with this condition throughout the year. Excessive coldness can effect skin color and appearance, posture and even confidence.

Blood circulation slows down during the colder months, and since your extremities are further from the heart, your heart has to work harder in winter to pump blood to these areas. Sometimes the vessels shrink when it is cold and the blood circulating back to the heart becomes weak.

Those with less active jobs (where they sit for prolonged periods of time) have a greater tendency to develop this condition than those with active jobs. Women are also more susceptible. Since men are naturally more yang, it is rare for men to suffer from this problem.

Those who have cold hands and a general cold feeling in the whole body throughout the year usually have a cold constitution and weak yang energy. These symptoms may be especially noticeable in late autumn and early spring. TCM offers some practical lifestyle recommendations, including keeping warm with appropriate clothing, self-massage, and soaking your hands and feet in herbal preparations such as a ginger or chili foot soak. Exercise such as running or ball sports can help to increase body temperature and improve circulation.

TCM also recommends the following foods:

- A tea can be made by adding two jujubes, three pieces of ginger (sliced) and 2 g of brown sugar to boiling water. Drink for one week. For those limiting sugar intake, omit or reduce the sugar.
- Onion and chili help those who have a cold constitution and always feel cold. Just add them to your food. Onions in particular improve circulation to the extremities.
- Cinnamon is beneficial for those with a cold constitution and yang deficiency. These people should increase warming foods, such as cinnamon, in their diet. Cinnamon can be consumed in food or as a tea.

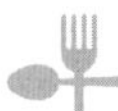

Warming Decoction to Improve Circulation

Ingredients: 6 g astragalus, 12 g parsnip, 6 g cinnamon stick, 250 ml water

Preparation:

1. Add astragalus, parsnip and cinnamon to water in a pot and boil for 20 minutes.
2. Strain and reserve the liquid in a container. Add new water to the pot and boil again for another 20 minutes.
3. Discard the herbs and add second liquid to the container with the first brew.
4. Drink twice a day, morning and afternoon.

2) Imbalance: Lymph Edema

Since the heart, small intestine, pericardium and *san jiao* meridians all travel through the arms, these meridians are fundamental for the function of the tendons and joints of the arms. Whenever there is stiffness, edema, pain or weakness, these meridians can be used in diagnosis and treatment. Treating edema will eliminate unsightly swelling.

External emedies for lymph edema: There are two points that can be used for edema of the arm, the Shenmen point and

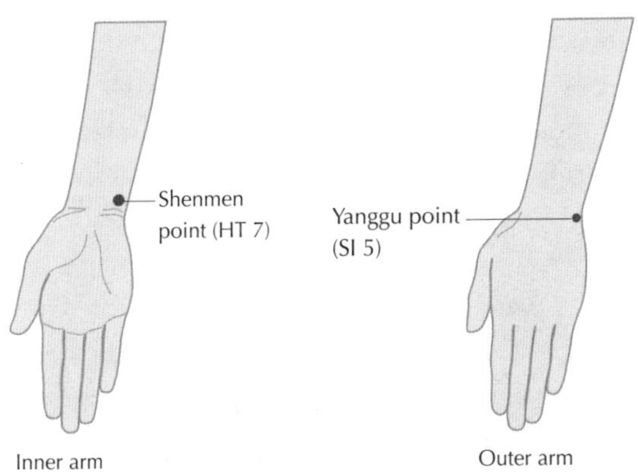

Fig. 39 Location of Shenmen point and Yanggu point

Yanggu point. You can massage these points yourself (fig. 39).

Lymph edema of the arms can also be caused by infection in the lymphatic system and glands. Another cause could be damage to the muscle close to the lymphatic system, which, in turn blocks circulation of lymph and causes arm swelling. In the case of filariasis, *tui na* (a special Chinese massage) and acupuncture to the meridians of the heart, small intestine, pericardium and *san jiao* can be used effectively to unblock stagnation and increase local blood flow to the area. Antibiotics may also be needed in the initial stages of the condition to kill the infection or parasite.

Additionally cancer and its treatments can sometimes lead to lymph edema. Radiotherapy itself can exasperate this condition, and the removal of lymph nodes, as sometimes occurs in cancer treatments, can also lead to a lot of swelling. Additionally the mental strain and inability to sleep during such a stressful life event, with the uncertainties and fear surrounding cancer, can worsen this condition. TCM is effective for helping to reduce the edema, and often activating the heart and urinary bladder meridians will be used to rebalance water metabolism and energy flow within these meridians.

Healthy Tongue

Maintaining healthy tongue function is important for normal and unimpeded speech, regular facial expression, and even optimal heart function. If these are compromised, confidence and appearance will be as well.

1) Imbalance: Speech Disorder

If the heart system cannot control the mind and mental activity, the tongue may become stiff and have small spasms. A simple example of this is when someone becomes nervous while giving a speech. The heart might start racing, and the person may also get sweaty palms, and become red faced and tongue-tied. When relaxed the symptoms disappear.

If someone has a speech disorder, a TCM doctor might use a lot of herbs and foods good for the heart system, and work on the meridians of the heart and pericardium to help improve speech issues. Clinical experience has shown this to be very effective, and has also developed some tongue exercises that help improve heart function.

2) Imbalance: Ulcers

If you begin to develop tongue ulcers it is your body's way of letting you know that you have to rebalance and reduce heart fire.

The following foods are recommended:

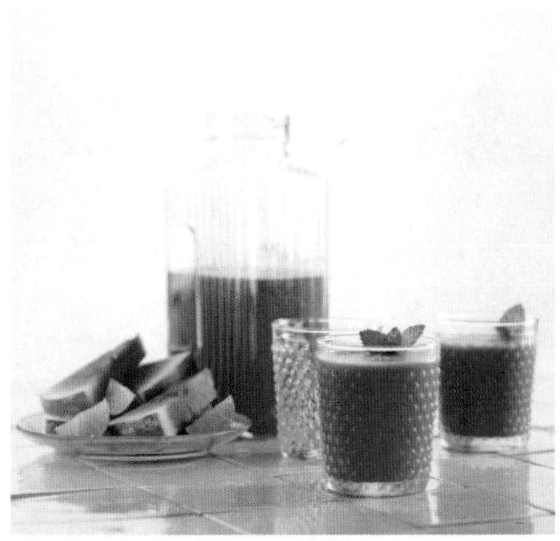

Fig. 40 Watermelon juice

1. You can drink watermelon juice (fig. 40), as it is cooling and soothing to a hot condition. Watermelon skin powder (*xi gua shuang*) is effective when applied locally on the ulcer. Wait a half hour before eating or drinking anything.

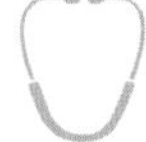

Treat Kidney for Ulcers

If the condition has set in and you have left it too long you may need to not only reduce heart fire but also strengthen the kidney and immune systems. Mulberry fruits are effective for tonifying the kidney. You can use 50 g fresh mulberry fruits or 15 g dried ones in a tea. Continue for three days.

Sound Sleep

The quality of your sleep is a good indicator of how your heart system is functioning. Sleep quality also affects your complexion.

We spend a fairly large proportion of our lives sleeping. In general, people spend one third of their lives asleep on average, although of course small children and elderly people sleep more. It is important to get seven to eight hours of sleep per night, though a small minority of people only need six or fewer hours.

People need to follow the earth's pattern. There is a saying in Chinese, *tian* (sky) *ren* (people) *xiang yin* (corresponding to each other), which means that during the day we should be awake and productive, and at night we should rest our body and allow the organ systems to recover. At night, your heart beat and breathing slow, and your blood pressure also changes. Your face, skin and hair detoxify and regenerate during the night.

It is especially important to go to sleep before 11 p.m. In TCM theory, sleeping between 11 p.m. and 3 a.m. is vital. This allows the liver and gall bladder to detoxify, and during this time, metabolism is regenerated.

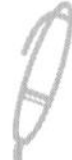

Five Leaf Gynostemma

Five leaf gynostemma (*jiao gu lan*) is also known as the poor man's ginseng. It goes to all five organ systems and can be useful for the prevention of tumors. It is an adephagan, helping with the growth, regeneration, and long life of the cells. In many regions of China known for longevity, it has been noted that this anti-aging herb is often consumed as a tea. It also helps to regulate and protect the liver, and can be useful in healing a fatty liver. It can reduce high lipids, and helps to contribute towards sound sleep and pain relief. This herb is nourishing for the liver blood. It is high in amino acids, vitamins, magnesium, iron, calcium, phosphorus, potassium, selenium, and zinc. It can be taken for 10–20 days and 100 g is usually a good dosage.

If you don't get good sleep between these hours, it will show up on your face and skin. When you are in your twenties it might not be noticeable, but as you get older, you might realize your face does not look refreshed if you miss out on quality sleep during that vital period. Working late into the night and a lack of sleep can age you prematurely, possibly leading to darkness under the eyes, pigmentation, liver spots, and rough or wrinkled skin.

1) Imbalance: Insomnia

The following foods are recommended:

- Gluey millet can be used to make a porridge, or you can use it in place of rice. There are also some lovely traditional snacks made with millet, peanuts and sugar. Almond milk with millet is another option.
- Asparagus lettuce (also called celtuce) can be eaten raw, juiced or stir-fried. Be sure to wash and peel the lettuce root (fig. 41).

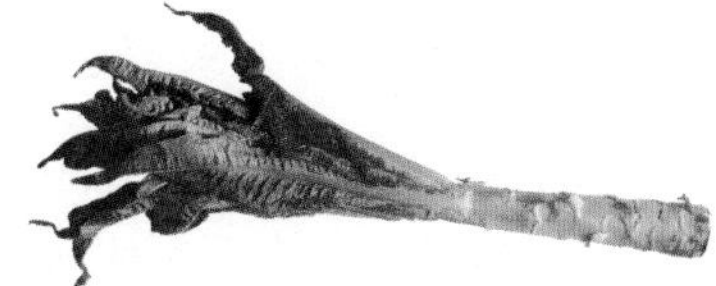

Fig. 41 Asparagus lettuce

2) Imbalance: Dream Disturbed Sleep

The following foods are recommended:

- Lingzhi mushroom is an effective tonic to promote sleep. In ancient times it was used as a tea or ground into a powder; now it can be bought in capsule form. Half an hour before bed, take between 0.5–1.5 g depending on your body weight, or if you are taking pharmacy-made lingzhi mushroom capsules then follow the prescribed dosage. Take for ten days, pausing for five days and then beginning a second course if necessary.
- Lily bulb clears heart heat and helps to promote a calm mind. It can relax the nerves and treat hysteria, and is

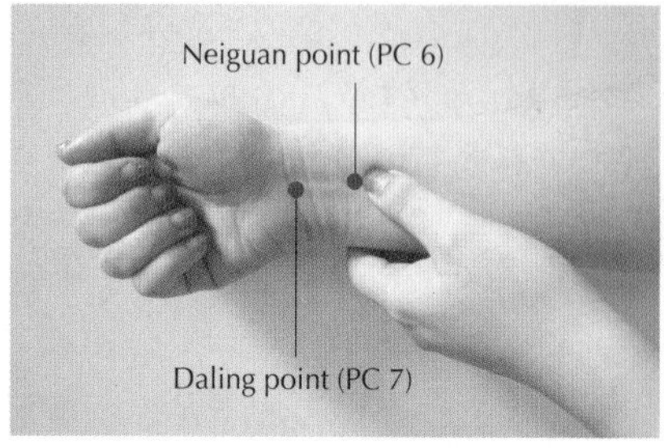

Fig. 42 Massage the Daling point and Neiguan point for sound sleep.

also effective for the relief of some types of dizziness. Including lily bulb in your diet can reduce anger, malaise and poor sleep disturbed by stressful dreams. Stir-fry 5 g fresh lily bulb with 50 g celery and six gingko nuts, consuming three times a week. You might also make a delicious tea, using 50 g lily bulbs and ten jujubes. If using dried lily bulbs you need to soak them for at least three hours, or preferably overnight. Add 300 g of water and cook for 20 minutes.

3) Imbalance: Sweaty Palms

When heart qi is insufficient, some of the following symptoms might be apparent: feeling nervous, not wanting to meet people, lacking confidence, feeling highly self-critical and overly afraid of other peoples' judgment, and sweaty palms. Heart qi deficiency might also cause sweaty palms in the summer even when someone does not feel nervous. Leaving symptoms untreated for prolonged periods of time can further weaken heart qi, so it is good to deal with it quickly.

This book does not address sweaty palms that are caused by a thyroid or genetic disorder. These remedies are applicable only for sweaty palms caused by an over reactive sympathetic nervous system.

There are many things that can be done to promote heart health and to correct imbalances, but most essential are a positive

Recipes for Excess Sweating

The following preparations can help heart qi to regulate the sympathetic nervous system in order to slow down or stop excess sweating.

Licorice root and rose bud tea. Place 10 g licorice root and 6 g rose buds in a cup. Add boiling water and drink as a tea. Use the same licorice root and rose buds throughout the day, refilling the boiling water three times per day. Drink for a 10-day period. Please note that those with high blood pressure need to use 10 g astragalus instead of licorice root, as licorice root can worsen high blood pressure.

American ginseng tea. Drink a tea containing 1 g of American ginseng every day for seven days.

Chinese angelica root tea. Angelica and astragalus are famous remedies for strengthening qi and blood. Angelica can promote rosy cheeks, regulate menstruation and clear out old blood. It can also tonify and regulate the blood while providing a remedy for sweaty palms caused by blood qi deficiency. It should not be used by people with a hot constitution or by people who have too much dampness in their bodies.

Dried oyster shell. Dried oyster shells can be made into a powder and taken as a tea. The powder can also be used topically, putting it on the hands to soak up excess sweat. After half an hour wash the powder off your hands.

outlook on life and a commitment to fostering happiness. Balancing your constitution and your yin and yang through food, tonics, acupressure, acupuncture and massage can also be important. Love your heart and it will show its appreciation with a glowing complexion, healthy blood vessels, good sleep, smooth circulation and ample nourishment for all your extremities.

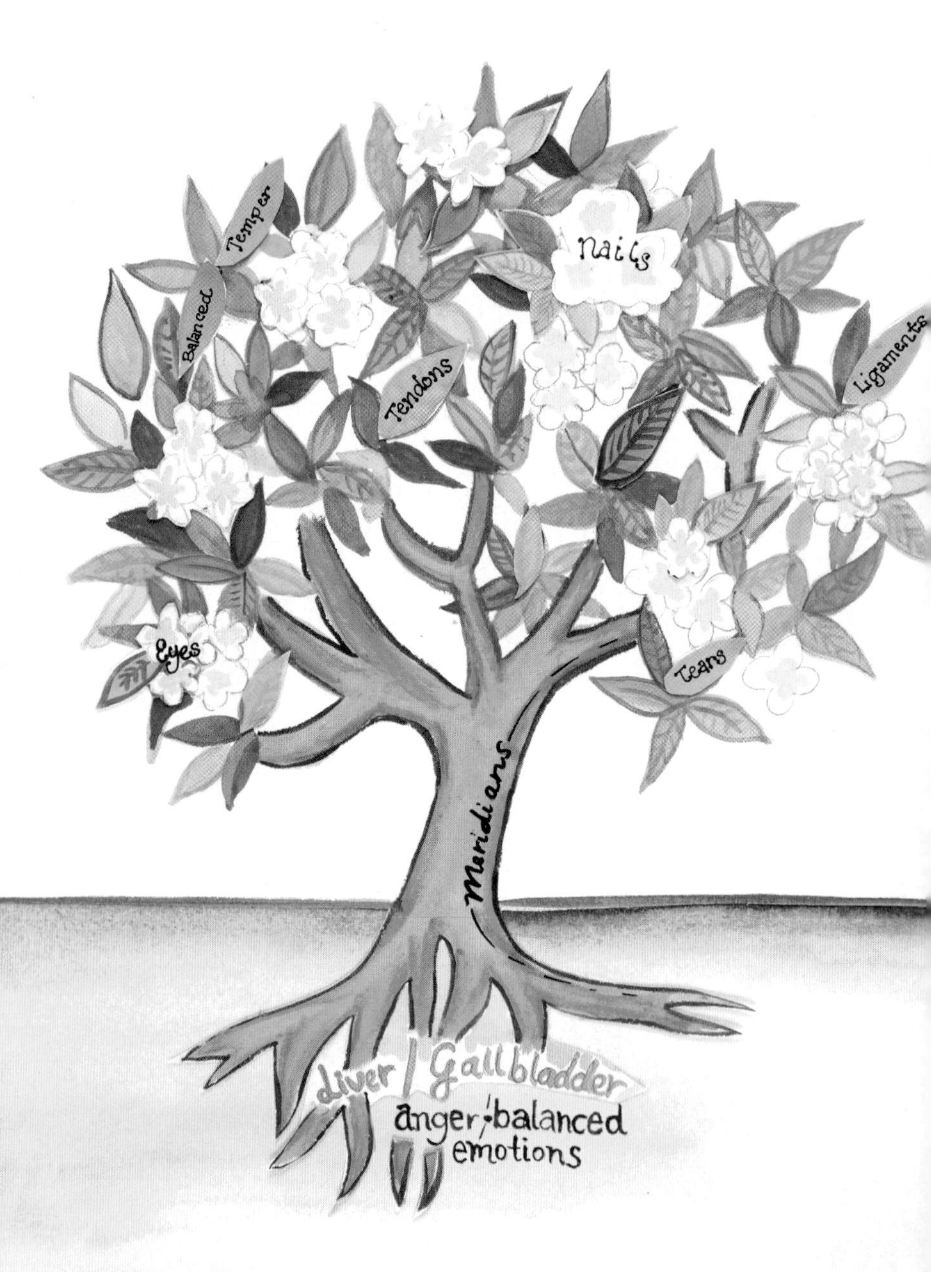
Temper
Balanced
Nails
Tendons
Ligaments
Eyes
Tears
Meridians
Liver / Gallbladder
anger/balanced
emotions

CHAPTER SIX
The Liver System

Roots

- *Zang*-organ: liver
- *Fu*-organ: gallbladder
- Emotion of anger

Trunk and Branches

- Meridians: Jueyin Liver Meridian of Foot, Shaoyang Gallbladder Meridian of Foot

Leaves

- Tears to moisten and protect the eyes
- Elastic, strong tendons and ligaments

Fruits

- Emotion of anger (also part of the "roots" system)

Flowers

- Clear, bright eyes
- Shiny, strong nails

Left Fig. 43 The liver system tree

1. Basic Facts about the Liver System

The liver system in traditional Chinese medicine includes the liver, gallbladder, and their meridian networks. It also includes the eyes, tears of the eyes, ligaments, and nails. The emotion related to this organ system is anger. While maintaining a balanced emotional state is dependent upon a strong liver system, being angry all the time can also be detrimental to it.

The liver has been described as the "general" of the body because it is the organ in charge of planning and mood regulation, including feelings of depression or excitement. A person, who is described as being courageous and determined, could also be described in Chinese medicine as a person with a strong liver.

The *Yellow Emperor's Canon* describes the liver as being responsible for strategy, and the gallbladder responsible for deciding whether or not the strategy is practical and applicable.

2. Functions of the Liver

Among its many important functions, the liver is responsible for storing blood and ensuring the smooth movement of qi throughout your entire system.

Regulating Qi for the Whole Body

The liver is responsible for ensuring a smooth flow of qi throughout the whole body and this impacts many of your biological functions. If qi is moving well, it will freely travel in upward and downward motions. This will facilitate blood circulation throughout the entire body and encourage the efficient movement of body fluid.

The positive relationship between qi, blood, and body

fluids is very important. Qi is yang, blood and body fluids are yin. When qi is moving in the right speed and direction and is not stagnated or disordered, then the blood and body fluids will follow suit.

The liver is also involved in ensuring that your qi is moving in the correct speed and directions. For instance, sometimes qi slows down and sinks. In this case, the liver helps it to go back upwards and disperse properly.

Working in close partnership with the heart, the liver plays a fundamental role in regulating all emotional activity. As you know, the heart controls the mind and spirit, and the mind and spirit help to govern your emotions. If the liver is able to adequately regulate the movement of qi, then we have balanced emotions and can respond to situations in a more positive way.

Furthermore, liver qi will aid healthy digestion, especially in relationship to absorption. A healthy liver will send nourishing essence to the gallbladder, which assists in the production of bile. In turn, the liver and gallbladder then work

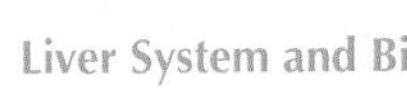

Liver System and Bile

If the liver is stagnated or liver's blood or yin is weak, it may not produce enough bile. Some people have a lot of bile so they don't experience any problems when eating a lot of meat, seeds, and nuts. Others struggle to create enough even if they are vegetarian or experience some digestive issues. With enough bile, constipation is less likely.

If the liver or gallbladder is imbalanced, a blockage of bile might occur. Some symptoms might include slow digestion with a yellow tinge to the skin. In this case, it is the bile needing another way to come out that causes the yellow coloration in the skin. Gallstones and/or a bitter taste in the mouth are other symptoms. Again the bitter taste is a result of bile coming up into the stomach rather than going down into the small intestine.

together to excrete bile into the small intestine in order to aid digestion. All bile is created as a result of the liver's nutrition, so bile excretion is dependent upon how much nourishing essence the liver can create.

Additionally, a strong liver with a smooth and consistent supply of liver qi will help to form a healthy reproductive system. This is pertinent for male ejaculation and the female menstrual cycle.

How can you determine whether the liver is adequately regulating qi?

To access how well your liver is regulating qi, a TCM doctor will pay attention to and ask you questions about certain areas of the body. These areas include: the top and sides of your head, the abdominal region (especially both sides of the lower abdomen, in line with the nipples and belly button), your groin area, both sides of your ribs and your tendons. The doctor may also enquire about and observe your eyes (how shiny they are, your vision, and any feelings you may have in your eyes such as pain, dryness or itchiness), and ask you about your mood including emotions such as unhappiness and anger.

When you have good liver function, qi will flow freely in the normal speed and directions. Your head and rib regions should be pain free. Your eyes will be shiny with sharp vision and your tendons will be flexible. Furthermore, outbursts or feelings of anger will not be a frequent occurrence.

Stagnation of liver qi will present with symptoms of bloating, feeling full,or distention in the above mentioned areas. Sighing often, sore breasts and eyes, and the avoidance of social situations may also be signs of liver qi stagnation.

Liver fire will cause a person to feel thirsty, hot, and sweat a lot. It may increase feelings of anger and a person may regularly have a red face and eyes.

Liver Stagnation

Liver stagnation occurs when liver qi is not flowing smoothly and becomes stuck or blocked.

The lower portions of the front of the ribcage including the 11th and 12th ribs and the tissue just below these ribs, should feel soft and smooth. However, these areas may feel hard and full when there is liver stagnation. Tenderness and/or fullness, and depression prior to menstruation. It's normal some breast swelling and tenderness may occur two to three days before menstruation, but any more than this could be a sign of liver stagnation.

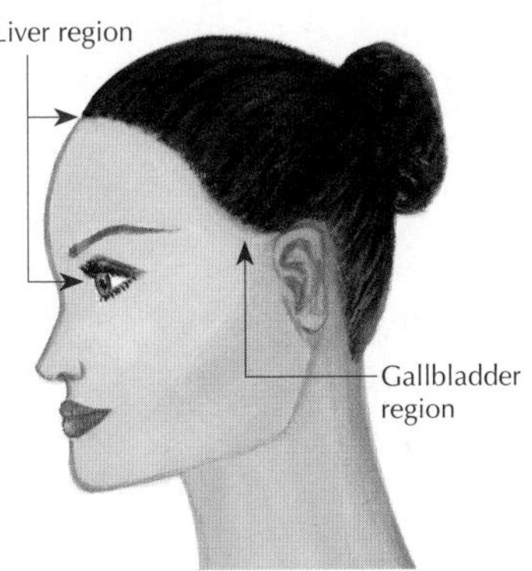

Fig. 44 The head area related to liver and gallbladder meridians

Migraines are another sign and the location of the migraine can bear some significance. Migraines will often appear on the sides of the forehead (which is known as the gallbladder region in TCM), the top of the head (liver region), and across the eyebrows (both liver and gallbladder regions) (fig. 44).

When liver stagnation is present, you may also get some fullness or tenderness on either side of the belly button or groin area ten days before menstruation. Furthermore, you might suffer from mood swings or depression.

For men, liver stagnation may show up as headaches, lack of sexual desire, prostate symptoms such as feelings of fullness or an enlarged prostate.

Liver Fire

Another commonly occurring liver imbalance is a condition known as liver fire. It is also called liver hyperactivity and occurs when there is too much yang in comparison to yin in the liver.

When a man has too much liver heat, he might feel hot often, perspire excessively, and have a constant thirst. He may become overly sexually active. Other accompanying signs may include aggression, anger, and the inclination to pick fights frequently. To remedy the symptoms caused by liver fire, he should participate in sports to rebalance the hyperactivity and excess liver heat.

For women, liver fire may present itself in pre-menstrual syndrome, including symptoms such as an explosive temper, aggression, violent outbursts, and yelling. In this case, there is too much liver yang that needs to be reduced to restore balanced emotions.

Cooling the heat/yang in the liver is important in bringing harmony to this situation. Both men and women might focus on finding ways to release their strong emotions to reduce the excess yang.

Food Therapy

Excess liver fire can be addressed by cooling the heat and much of this can be done through dietary choices.

Lifestyle Adjustment

Those with an overriding cold constitution may not want to have too many "cold" or "cooling" foods in their diet. In this case, liver yang can be reduced with lifestyle choices such as engaging in an enjoyable hobby, participating in sports, finding a way to sweat, and talking about your feelings. If you don't have anyone to talk to, writing down your feelings might provide a sense of relief.

Massage

Massage could also help because the oil can encourage excess heat to come out through the pores of the skin. These are better options for those with an underlying cold constitution and for those with "cold stomach" conditions rather than the over consumption of cooling foods. Those with a cold stomach may also use acupuncture and swimming to feel less angry.

Nourish the Blood

Women should also incorporate strategies to nourish the blood. Nourishing the blood, which is yin, is an important approach for women since they lose large amounts during menstruation and it needs to be replaced. By bringing the levels of blood back to normal, this yin substance effectively counterbalances the excess yang. Therefore this re-establishes the yin-yang balance in the liver. Actually, the process of losing blood during menstruation also helps to remove surplus liver yang. This is why the symptoms of PMS are often relieved once menstruation arrives. Childbirth is another way for women to reduce liver yang so women have two in-built strategies for reducing this condition. The only strategy for men is ejaculation.

Increase Yin

Another strategy is to rebalance yang is by increasing yin. Yin weakness also produces more yang, according to TCM. Evidence of this is dry mouth, thirst, night sweats, nervousness, and restlessness. So creating a time for quiet or relaxation is vital for nourishing body fluid and yin.

Not everyone is this constitutionally complicated and those who have an underlying yang/heat condition can easily increase cooling foods within their diet. As mentioned, some people have mixed symptoms and may need the assistance of a TCM practitioner who will combine therapies in order to re-establish balance.

Storing and Directing Blood

The liver plays a role in storing blood and directs the blood to different areas of the body as we need it, according to TCM theory.

Blood is produced in the body by several organs. Once you are asleep, the blood will be stored in the liver for detoxing and regeneration.

Blood is available for use wherever it is needed. And the liver will direct the blood to different areas of the body. For example, when we study, or require a lot of mental energy, the liver directs blood to our head so we can think clearly. When we participate in sports, the liver sends blood to the limbs and muscles so that our body has adequate blood flow to take action. This blood flow is important for ensuring the joints and ligaments are well nourished and lubricated.

The liver stores blood not only for the whole body, but also for itself. The quantity of blood stored in the liver needs to be sufficient for a balance of yin-yang, which is essential for:

- The formation of basic instincts such as appetite for food and sexual desire. The liver is the most important organ for regulating qi, storing blood, and ensuring the body has enough blood. It also regulates stomach and reproductive rhythms. The blood volume in the liver is highly relevant to all kinds of physical activities.

- Preventing liver hyperactivity. Blood is yin, and having enough blood stored in your liver is essential to balance and house the yang. According to yin-yang theory, yin and yang can help and control each other. When one becomes weak, the other can become too strong causing disharmony. If your body does not have enough yin (blood and body fluid), then the yang might become overpowering and this may result in a person feeling simultaneously weak, hot and impatient.
- Managing emotional health. The liver is the "general" of the body and has a major influence on your emotional state of being. It has a strong influence on your qi's conduction, dispersion, and blood storage. Therefore, it has a special relationship to the emotional state of the whole body, not just anger.

When we discuss terms such as the liver has inadequate blood, it is important to remember that we are speaking from a Chinese medical perspective, not a Western medical viewpoint. The liver not having enough blood sounds like a serious medical condition from a Western medical model. Though in TCM, it

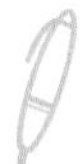

The Formation of Blood

The stomach, spleen, kidney, and heart are all involved with blood production. The formation of blood comes from two sources. The first being acquired essence that is created as a result of the nutrition we assimilate and absorb, and the second being our stored kidney essence.

The spleen and stomach break down nutrients from food through the digestion process. Our body then produces nutrition qi and body fluids. These two basic materials travel through the heart and lung, and eventually produce red colored blood.

This is how food essence is transformed into blood and why Chinese medicine often addresses anemia by strengthening the spleen, stomach, and kidney. This is so acquired essence is available for transformation into iron rich blood.

makes reference to minor imbalances that are occurring and can be adjusted fairly easily with food choices, herbs, acupuncture, or other TCM modalities. Likewise, by making minor adjustments as you become aware of a certain imbalance, you can greatly improve the health of your liver and ultimately also affect your physical appearance.

3. Meridians of the Liver System

The gallbladder and liver meridians cooperate together to circulate qi, blood and body fluids. These meridians are found on the trunk of the body, neck, and on the legs.

The Jueyin Liver Meridian of Foot (fig. 45) begins from the big toe close to the nail and travels up on top of the foot between the first and second toe. It then moves up on the inside of the

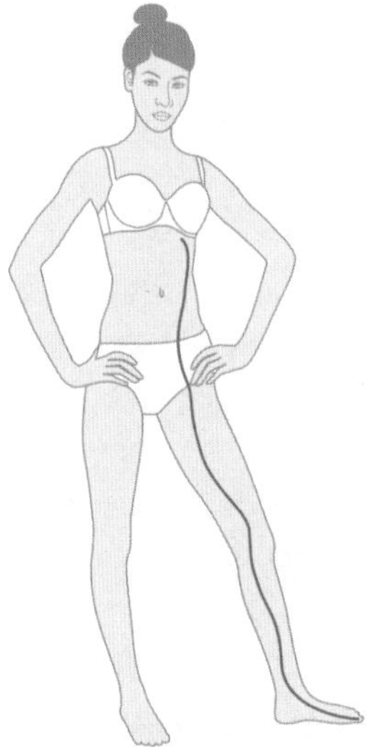

Fig. 45 The Jueyin Liver Meridian of Foot

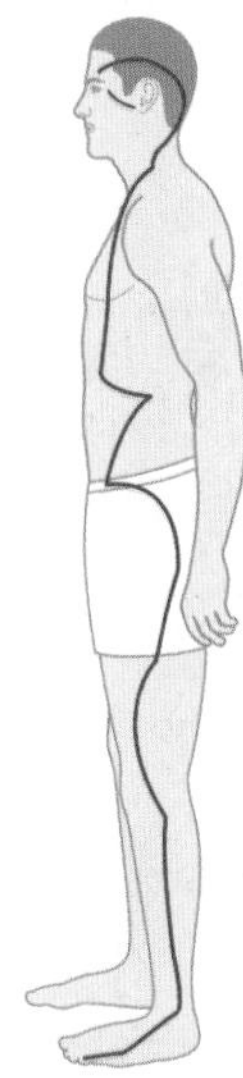

Fig. 46 Shaoyang Gallbladder Meridian of Foot

leg, inside the thigh, across the groin and circles the reproductive area. From here, it passes the waist to the front of the lower ribs. Internally, it travels around the deep stomach points then circles the gallbladder organ, over the diaphragm, and zig zags the region beneath the rib area, and up to the breast, eyes and top of head. Since this book is mainly for beauty, we only use less detailed meridian pictures.

The Shaoyang Gallbladder Meridian of Foot starts from the Taiyang point (Temple point), travels across on the top of the head, behind of the eyes and ears, and then to the backs of the shoulders, down the side of the trunk, hips, legs, and ankles, ending outside the fourth toe (fig. 46).

4. Liver System and Beauty

With so much emphasis on outward appearance, it can be easy to take for granted the impact a healthy liver system has on our beauty.

Eyes and Tears: Window and Liquid of the Liver

According to the *Yellow Emperor's Canon*, "the liver nourishes the blood so that we can have clear vision." This famous book goes on to say that, "When liver qi is flowing smoothly, the eyes can identify five colors."

In Chinese medicine, the eyes are linked to the liver via meridians. The liver controls the eyes so looking after your liver can help you have beautiful and memorable eyes. Dull and emotionless eyes are not so attractive. Whereas, eyes that are expressive and full of life can form powerful connections.

Very happy, optimistic, and energetic people often have a sparkle in their eyes that can be very appealing. Those eyes may even have the power to capture someone's heart. Furthermore, bright and vibrant eyes are highly valued as a sign of good health

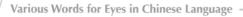

Various Words for Eyes in Chinese Language

When talking about eyes, Chinese people may use different terms depending on the context of the conversation. There have been many poems written describing lovely eyes as deep, shiny pools.

目 (*mu*): The ancient Chinese term for eyes. It is still used today particularly in idioms, proverbs, and poems.

精明 (*jing ming*): This word means essence and spirit. The essence from each of the five organs provides basic building blocks that contribute to the structural materials of the eyes and ensures their healthy function. The saying "the eyes are the window to the soul" reflects the idea that the eyes are expressive and can communicate a lot about the soul of a person.

眼睛 (*yan jing*): In modern times, this term is used both in anatomical and everyday language.

in virtually every culture.

The eyes should be clear, shiny, and have enough liquid to create a reflection, according to TCM. In traditional Chinese culture, eyes were often observed to judge someone's cleverness. Bright, clear, and alert eyes (switched on, so to speak) not only were an indication that the person was clever, but also that he or she was healthy enough to enable a state of focus, consciousness, and awareness.

Traditionally and in the present day, yellow coloration in the eyes can be an indication that the fine essence is not coming up adequately and a sign that the eyes are literally aging. It can also be a sign that the liver is having trouble detoxifying. This may be due to liver heat and dampness decreasing the liver's detoxification functions and causing toxins to build up, which is ultimately reflected in the eyes.

The liver plays a crucial role in creating tears, according to TCM. The passage between the eyes and the nose needs good water circulation. This provides moisture to allow a full range of eye movement. This water is also essential for shiny eyes since it creates a reflection to make the eyes appear shiny. Less water or inefficient circulation of water in the eyes causes this shine to decrease. Chinese people highly value glistening eyes and have two phrases regarding this. *"Shui ling ling"* describes good circulation of water inside of the eyes that results in enough moisture to nourish and protect them. However, there is not too much causing consistently watery or teary eyes. The other phrase is *"shui wang wang"*, which means there is enough water to make the eyes shine and reflect the light resulting in beautiful and memorable eyes. Observing the vitality of the eyes is a diagnostic tool in TCM.

Breasts: Outer Territory of the Liver

Since both the liver and stomach meridians cross over the breast, issues with the liver may manifest in the breasts. If a young woman is late in developing breasts during puberty, a TCM doctor might address liver and kidney function. During adulthood, supporting and balancing liver and stomach function are often very effective in creating beautiful healthy breasts.

Breast health begins at puberty. Girls as young as 10–12 years old can begin to influence the health and appearance of their breasts. At this time, the harmonization of the liver and kidney system initiates the growth of breasts at puberty.

At age 14, the kidney essence becomes full for girls and they will begin to excrete sexual development hormones. These hormones cause the stomach and liver meridian to open up and also help to carry nutrition needed in the breast area. At this time, the liver's blood becomes enriched and the liver meridian become more smooth and regulated in the breast area causing the breasts to grow. If liver essence or blood is slow to develop, then breast growth can become postponed.

Menstruation should begin one or two years after breast development. Menstruation helps expel toxins and assists the regeneration of the lining of the uterus during each monthly cycle. At the beginning of their menstruation, young girls may find that their cycles are a bit irregular, but this should settle down after the first two years. Breasts continue to develop and are boosted by estrogen, which is one of the hormones produced as a result of a healthy menstrual cycle.

The nipple and breast areas are internally and externally related to the liver, stomach, gallbladder, and the meridians. Illnesses of the breasts have a close relationship with fast food, disharmony of the internal emotions, and weight gain. All of these symptoms can be linked back to these organs. A treatment program may require addressing all of them.

Tendons: Tissue of the Liver

Each organ system is paired with a body tissue via its meridians and the tissue of the liver system is the tendons. Tendons link muscles to joints and bones. They have a small and restricted range of elasticity, and help to facilitate a full range of motion while keeping the joint stable.

The tendons are dependent upon liver qi and the liver meridians to bring nourishing blood from the liver. If the liver qi or meridians are not functioning optimally and do not supply enough nourishing blood, tendons may become dehydrated and this may affect their function. If someone is constantly spraining his or her tendons, it may be a sign that the liver qi is not flowing smoothly or that the liver's blood is insufficient.

Certain symptoms may be present if the liver has a blood deficiency and the tendons are also lacking adequate nutrition. These include numbness in the legs or arms, lack of coordination in the joints, and rigid movements when attempting to contract and release muscles. Furthermore, a straight and upright posture when sitting or walking can indicate that the liver is providing enough blood and qi to your tendons and ligaments for them to function optimally. Balanced liver yin and yang is important for a great posture. Those who get tired easily and cannot maintain an upright posture, even when they know it is good to do so, may have an imbalance in the liver organ system.

Nails: Flower of the Liver

Healthy nails, including fingernails and toenails, should be strong, flexible, shiny, hydrated, with a pink color visible beneath the surface of the nail bed.

Nails are the extension of the tendons, just as the teeth are the extension of the bones in the kidney system, according to Chinese medicine.

If your nails are strong, then it is likely that you have a healthy liver system with enough nourishment being assimilated, produced, and then circulated to support your whole liver system. If your nails are weak and not growing quickly, it might be an indication that your liver is generating inadequate nourishment to support each element of the liver system. Your nails, the last in the chain to receive this nourishment, might suffer if you are not generating good liver qi, blood, and circulation.

Weak brittle nails might be communicating a message to you about the health of your liver system.

Thin nails with dry areas that lack shine, or nails that have a purple or pale color to them, might indicate liver blood deficiency or poor circulation.

Dry areas on the nails and vertical lines can also indicate the same condition. Alternatively, the liver may have enough blood, but because stagnation is present, it compromises the liver's ability to bring nourishing blood to the nail bed. This leads to nails that are not optimally healthy.

Some TCM doctors believe that your nails should have the ability to breath (just as the skin does), and since the liver opens up to the nails via meridians, covering the nails with polish can inhibit this process. Wearing nail polish too often, or nail polish of inferior quality is not recommend. Of course, never wearing nail polish might seem a bit boring. Even TCM doctors who recommend avoiding nail polish agree that wearing it on special occasions is acceptable as long as you give your nails the opportunity to breath more often than not.

Another factor about nail polish is that it contain some toxins. Some TCM doctors believe that these toxins can be absorbed through the nails and into the liver meridians, eventually being absorbed by the liver. We should understand that whatever is placed on our skin or nails can be absorbed by the body, ultimately making its way to the liver. But TCM adds another dimension to this thought with the discussion of meridians.

Skin Color Changes: Signal of Liver Toxin

In TCM theory, pigmentation on the skin such as brown, red spider dots, or red palm is a signal of accumulated toxins in your liver system. Toxins, in the TCM context, refer to excess conditions such as stagnation, heat, fire, and damp-heat invading the liver. There are many different kinds of pigmentation that can occur on the skin and we will provide a brief outline of some of them below:

- Birthmarks. The larger lighter type of pigmentation that is found usually, but not limited to, the upper legs or lumber area on the back. Other commonly occurring birthmarks are small dark or beige spots that can be found anywhere on the body. Some birthmarks might change, becoming more raised and grow hair in times when we are too exhausted and stressed, but are usually not dangerous. These types of pigmentation are usually congenital.
- Benign and cancerous moles. We will not be addressing remedies for benign or cancerous moles in this book.
- Using too many antibiotics too often can cause liver blood stagnation, which manifests in brown pigmentation.

Generally speaking, the pigmentation can dispel once you stop using the antibiotics, especially if you help to nourish and regulate the liver blood circulation and qi movements.

- Liver spots and brown pigmentation during or after pregnancy and menopause. It is a result of changing hormones and weakened kidney essence during these periods of life. They are also related to liver dysfunction.
- White spots that lack pigmentation can be caused by having a blood deficiency of the liver.

Face pigmentation, if caused by liver blood stagnation, is usually accompanied by symptoms of dark and clotted menstrual blood, painful menstruation, or a purple tongue. This pattern is often caused by stagnation of liver qi. When qi stagnates, it eventually causes blood to also stagnate. Since the liver stores blood, it is particularly affected by this condition.

Toxins can come into our body through our environment, food, water, and the air we breathe. If our organ systems are strong, we can usually deal efficiently with these toxins. Those with a weak liver system may be susceptible to liver qi stagnation could particularly if they have strong emotional responses to their environment or to something that has happened. Liver qi stagnation could leads to blood stagnation, food stagnation, damp-stagnation, and phlegm stagnation. All of these conditions can lead to other illnesses.

It is important to detoxify the liver before it becomes overwhelmed and address qi stagnation before the other types of stagnation begin to set in. Other organs, like the lung and spleen can also help to remove food, phlegm, and damp stagnation and may be also treated if these conditions are present.

Anger: Emotion of the Liver

The emotion related to the liver is anger, including suppressed anger or violent anger.

If a person demonstrates regular out-bursts of anger, for no apparent reason, and seems grumpy all the time, there may be some underlying liver dysfunction that needs addressing. Feeling angry often could be a result of liver heat or liver yin, and blood deficiency. A TCM doctor would address this by reducing liver heat or fire, and strengthening the liver blood or yin.

When liver yin and yang is out of balance, the unhealthy anger will appear in our life. Being constantly angry can cause harm to the liver and ultimately lead to further dysfunction:

- It may cause liver yang to become hyperactive and can create a myriad of symptoms.
- It may cause a lot of toxins to build up in the body. These toxins can make you more prone to wrinkles and pigmentation.
- Biological chemicals produced as a result of anger can get stuck in the skin producing a dull, yellow, and gloomy complexion. They can also affect digestion, your nervous and cardiovascular systems, and your ability to think clearly. Furthermore, chronic anger affects the immune system and can make you more susceptible to chronic inflammation, which is aging to the body.
- Additionally, you are strengthening the muscles that pull your face in a downward motion when you frown. Constantly frowning can pull your face in a direction you may not want it to go, causing expression lines and a tendency towards sagging especially after middle age.

5. Beauty Problems and Enhancement

Now we will discuss four beauty concerns that are related to your liver system and provide some food options and herbal recipes that will benefit your liver.

It is wise to deal with imbalances when you first notice them and before they become a major issue.

If you cannot seem to rebalance your system and relieve your symptoms using the natural and food remedies provided, you might seek treatment by seeing a TCM doctor who can help unblock stagnation of liver qi, restore yin-yang balance, and help the qi move a lot faster.

The taste associated with the liver is sour. Sour foods help to regulate the liver and ensure liver function is smooth and effective. If you want to help detoxify your liver, you could include a sour citrus fruit such as grapefruit.

Enticing Eyes

Since qi and blood is carried up through the liver meridian to the eyes, many eye conditions are a result of the liver system getting out of balance. Therefore, many eye conditions can be treated by addressing the liver.

One way to regulate the liver and support eye function is to massage the liver and gallbladder meridians. Actually, the kidney also works together with the liver and plays a role in creating vibrant eyes, according to TCM. Furthermore, the kidney helps to create lovely eyelashes and brows, which frame the eyes.

1) Imbalance: Red Eyes

When the liver has too much heat, the eyes may become red, accompanied by a burning sensation or a feeling that there is a foreign body inside the eye. Cloudy vision and possibly visible clouding in the eye itself are other signs that liver heat may be present. There may or may not be discharge as well. Two common imbalances that often affect the eyes are "damp heat" and "wind heat".

Damp heat: May cause bacterial eye infections, symptoms such as red eyes, dull pain in the eyes, eye discharge (sometimes

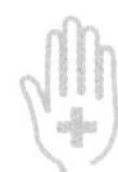

Eye Massage

If performed regularly, it can really improve the appearance of your eyes, reduce wrinkles, and lift the eyes. The massage can be done with or without face oil.

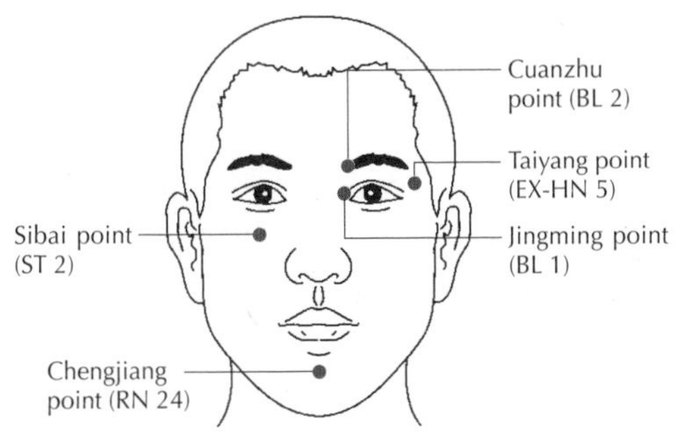

Fig. 47 Acupoints for eye massage

How to Apply?

1.Sit still with your ankle, knees, hips all at right angle, or lie down in a comfortable position. In these positions energy from your *dan tian* can easily be sent up to your eyes.

2.Find the Cuanzhu point using the tip of your thumbs. Massage in circular motions 32 times clockwise and 32 times anticlockwise (fig. 47).

3.Inside the depression against the bridge of the nose in line with the inner eye, find the next Jingming point to massage. Repeat the procedure of massaging the point for a total of 64 circles.

4.The next Sibai point are just below your eyes (in line with your eyeballs on the peaks of the cheekbones). Find a small depression and use your index fingers to repeat the massage procedure, you can rest your thumbs on the jaw.

5.Place the thumbs on the side of the temple (Taiyang point) and use the outer edge of the forefingers to massage across the eyebrows (starting from the inside out and moving in straight lines). Alternate between the top of the eyebrows and the bone under the eyes (also from the inside out). Then follow the same path to massage in small circles.

yellow in color), allergies, tearful eyes, sensitivity to light, or yellow coloration in the whites of your eyes.

Wind heat: May cause hay fever, which can be accompanied by itchy, watery, and swollen eyes. Redness in the eyes in the season of spring or summer, which has been caused by allergies, can be diagnosed according to either wind heat or damp heat.

Distinguishing whether your symptoms are attributed to damp or wind heat can be a little complicated, but symptoms of wind heat include less discharge accompanied by more red, watery, and itchy eyes. Damp heat, on the other hand, bears symptoms of more swelling, pain, and yellow discharge.

The following foods are recommended:

- Chamomile is a cooling herb that is excellent for the liver heat and eye conditions. You can drink it as a tea and apply the teabags to your eyes. Place them on your eyes after soaking the teabags for a minute in boiling water and then allowing them to cool down. By drinking chamomile tea and applying the teabags as an eye pack, you can achieve very effective results and can even treat a sty in the early stages.
- Those with a cold constitution might have eye discharge that is less yellow or even whitish. These people may do well consuming leek to remove wind heat. The season of spring often brings with it viruses and the accompanying winds of spring can spread these viruses more rapidly.

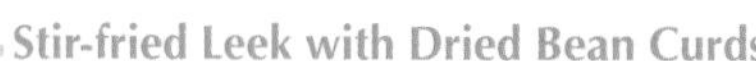

Stir-fried Leek with Dried Bean Curds

In China, stir-fried leek with dried bean curds is a traditional dish often cooked in spring time to prevent eye infections that are caused by spring wind and heat.

Ingredients: 200 g of leek, and three pieces of dried bean curds

How to Prepare?

1. Cut 200 g of leek and three pieces of dried bean curds into bite size pieces.
2. Heat 5 g of vegetable oil and stir-fry the dried bean curds for the first ten seconds.
3. Add the leek, 3 g of salt and stir-fry for another two minutes.

- Cassia seeds are believed to be anti-bacterial and can help improve blurry vision caused by cataracts. They can reduce night blindness and are effective in eliminating redness in the eyes caused by pink eye or the flu. These seeds are very good for cooling the liver and causing the eyes to shine. Make a tea using one teaspoon of whole or powdered cassia seeds. Please note that cassia seeds have a laxative effect and are not suited to those with loose bowel movements, an aversion to cold drinks, or a weak stomach. If you get diarrhea or watery stools, you might use celery or celery seeds instead.

2) Imbalance: Itchy Eyes

Itchy, red eyes and seasonal allergies can be related back to the liver and can be treated effectively using liver supporting foods, treatments, and herbs. Wind heat is a common cause for itchy eyes. However, it could indicate a blood or body fluid weakness if the symptoms are prolonged.

The following foods are recommended:

- To treat wind heat, you can consume celery (parsley), which is very good for liver function, regulating allergy reactions, expelling wind, and stopping the itchiness.

Celery Juice

Recipe 1: Create a celery juice using enough stalks to make 60–100g of juice. Celery juice by itself tastes rather bland.

Recipe 2: A combination of apple, celery, and carrot juice is much more appetizing and the carrot and celery juices together will both target the liver meridian. Apple is good to tonify yin. Yin deficiency can present with symptoms of regular thirst, night sweats, and dryness. Adding an apple a day can be very good for those with these symptoms.

Recipe 3: If you have a cold stomach, then you might add a little piece of ginger (or a few drops of ginger juice). Although this juice combination is generally not too cooling in nature.

Celery (parsley) is pungent and therefore very effective for expelling wind. You could eat it raw or add it to your juice. You might also add it to the top of your food, such as in a fish dish. It would not only garnish, but function as a pungent liver regular.

- Itchy eyes can also helped by drinking mint tea. Drinking 5 g of mint leaves with 5 g of Flos Eriocauli (*gu jing cao*) can make your eyes shine and can also remove the feeling of having a foreign body in the eye.
- Five grams of mulberry leaf, with 5 g of parsnip can be consumed as a tea to enrich body fluid and counteract dryness. This is also an effective remedy to expel wind heat and treat itching, red, swollen eyes.

3) Imbalance: Yellow Eyes

Clear whites of the eyes shows that your blood is harmonized and clear. Early stages of jaundice, or conditions of high cholesterol may produce a yellow color on the inner whites of the eyes (closest to the nose).

What is now known as high cholesterol was referred to in ancient times as a blocked vessel with dampness or phlegm and checking this region of the eyes can help with detection of this condition.

The following foods are recommended:

- Chicory, both the root and leaf, is also very good for the liver and gallbladder. Chicory root is in the same family as chrysanthemum and is also cooling in temperature and slightly bitter. It is effective for removing heat and water retention, and can help to reduce swelling and heat in the eyes. It can effectively reduce or treat yellow eye discharge and yellow coloring in the whites of the eyes. In many restaurants in China, chicory leaves are used as a starter to a meal and are combined with a little olive oil and vinegar.

- Chrysanthemum leaf is the sprout of the chrysanthemum. Since it is cooling in nature, it can be used effectively to treat sensitivity to hot seasons.
- Gardenia (*zhi zi*) is cold in nature and bitter in taste. Its function is to remove toxins and fire, expel dampness and heat, cool the blood, and simulate blood circulation. Use 50 g fresh gardenia or 9 g dry gardenia to treat yellow eyes and urine. Combining the previous dose with 6 g of artemisia capillaris (*yin chen hao*) is very effective for treating acute hepatitis A and cholecystitis with symptoms of fever, yellow eyes, skin, and urine.

4) Imbalance: Dry Eyes

Tears are responsible for protecting and nourishing the eyes. Dry eyes (in need of eye drops) occur when the eyes do not produce enough tears. Dry eyes may be accompanied by blurred or weak vision, such as night blindness. They might also be accompanied by the feeling of having a foreign body inside the eye or feeling tired after reading for a short time (unrelated to vision problems). These symptoms may be diagnosed as liver yin and blood deficiency. Yin (including blood and body fluids) is needed to provide moisture for your tears.

Blurred vision combined with dizziness can be caused by a liver yin deficiency with an empty heat. An empty heat is created when there is a deficiency of liver yin (body fluids) and presents itself with symptoms of hotness, usually in the afternoon or early evening. A red face may accompany it along with five palm heat (palms, souls of feet and chest), hot flushes, and sweat. To remedy this kind of blurred vision and dry eyes, you should focus on tonifying the body fluids instead of aggressively trying to reduce heat.

The following foods are recommended:

- Shiitake mushrooms are very good for the liver and can

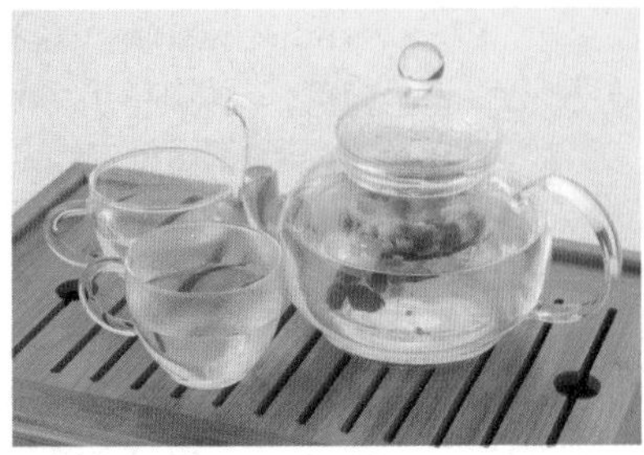
Fig. 48 Chrysanthemum and wolfberries tea

help to remove phlegm and toxins from this important organ. They are neutral in nature, neither too cooling nor heating for the body, and are effective for enhancing liver energy and strength. The dried shiitake mushrooms contains no fungus and are a great alternative for people who have candida or an allergy to fungus. Those who begin to experience symptoms in moldy conditions should choose dried shiitake mushrooms instead of fresh ones. Those who do not suffer with these conditions should choose the fresh ones when they are available. Five grams of dried shiitake mushrooms or 10 g of fresh ones is a good dosage.

- Chrysanthemum and wolfberries are a very famous pair in China and are often consumed as a tea together. They are excellent in treating liver heat and can help reduce feelings of hotness in summer or during menopause. They can also be used to help combat mental stress (fig. 48).

Other foods that can help with eye conditions include: mulberry, blackberry, and green apple. Eating these fruits will nourish the liver and strengthen the body fluids. Most of these foods have a sour sweet taste, which is good for regenerating body fluids. The juice from these fruits will help to produce fluids that will nourish the yin within your blood stream. In turn, this will help to remove dryness, blurred vision, and will ultimately improve the shine in your eyes. Besides the fact that raspberry is a warming fruit and mulberry has cooling properties, they are both successful in helping the liver. Raspberry is a liver, kidney, and yang tonic.

Beautiful Breasts

Some people carry a lot of stress in their breast tissue. For instance some women do not adapt to stress in their early 20's and do not take care of the food they eat. As a result, they carry blockages later in life in their breast tissue.

Comfort foods are often chosen in periods of stress. In the West, these may include chocolates, wine, cookies, and ice cream. In China, glutinous rice, sweet dumplings, azuki bean powder, Chinese pudding with jujubes, and longan are chosen.

For cleansing the breasts, do a regular self-massage and breast stretching.

Reducing anger and increasing your intake of food known to improve breast conditions such as cysts and solid nodules is another important strategy.

1) Imbalance: Slow Development or Sagging Breasts

Slow development of the breasts during puberty, sagging, and early aging of the breasts can be addressed using natural methods. Sagging occurs when the breast tissue begins to break down.

In China, it is common for people to do two things to combat these conditions. The first is applying a warm pack (wheat pack or a warm wet towel) then massaging the breasts in order to help draw blood circulation to the area. The second strategy, which can also help the breast become fuller and more elastic, is a rice wine and chicken egg recipe.

The following foods are recommended:

- Beef, pork, or mutton tendons can improve breast fullness. In China, tendons are very easy to find, but you may need to make a special request to your local butcher outside of China.

- If you are not a fan of eating tendons, then you can use dried bamboo fungus (*zhu sun*) to achieve a similar result. Bamboo fungus is known to make your skin very tender. It is high in protein and is also very high in zinc, iron and magnesium. It is renowned in China as a beauty food

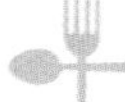

Rice Wine and Chicken Egg

Ingredients: water, 1 egg, rice wine 50 g (It can be found in Asian supermarkets and will usually have some rice pieces floating in it.)

How to Prepare?

1. Boil 500 ml of water.
2. Add one beaten egg, cook for five minutes.
3. Add 50 g rice wine. When you add the wine, the water will appear to stop boiling momentarily; allow it to reach boiling point again, then immediately turn off the stove.
4. Add some honey or maple syrup to sweeten in moderation or eat with something sweet like cookies or chocolate three days before menstruation to encourage well-formed breasts.

Dried Bamboo Fungus Soup

Ingredients: dried bamboo fungus 10 g, mushroom 30 g, peas 50 g, carrots 50 g, salt 3 g, olive oil 5 g, water 1L

How to Prepare?

1. Soak the dried bamboo fungus in room temperature water for 20 minutes.
2. Clean and chop the bamboo fungus, mushroom and carrots into bite size pieces.
3. Add water, peas and carrots to a pan or an earth-wear pot. Bring to the boil and stew for five minutes.
4. Then add the bamboo fungus. After three minutes, add the mushroom and bring it to boil again. Add salt and oil and turn off the heat.

Dried bamboo fungus can also be turned into a stock. It is very nice when combined with coriander, green vegetables, or pumpkin. Bamboo fungus can also be added to chicken soup.

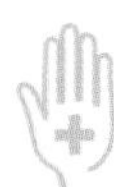

How to Apply Breast Self-Massage?

The following massage can be very helpful or healthier and more beautiful breasts. It can:

- Bring circulation, energy, and body fluids to the breast area
- Open up certain local acupuncture points and meridians on and around the breasts
- Remove blockages and stagnation
- Develop firm, lovely breasts for young girls
- Prevent sagging after breast-feeding
- Prevent lumps and blockages

How to Apply?

1. Either have a warm bath, shower, or use a hot towel to warm the breast area.

2. Massage the Danzhong Point with the thumb or fingertips in small clockwise circles for 20 seconds (fig. 49).

3. Massage the Zhongfu point with the middle finger in circular motions for 20 seconds. Use the left middle finger to massage the right side point and the right middle finger to massage the left side point.

4. Pinch the pectoral muscle with a short, gentle pumping action. Put the thumb on the Zhongfu point and the rest fingers deep into the armpit. Use the left hand to massage the right muscle and right hand to massage the left muscle. This regulates the lymph, stimulates blood circulation, and helps to release stagnation and blockages.

5. Using all of your fingers, massage the root of the breasts where they attach to the ribs. If you have larger breast, you may need to use two hands. Gently pump the breasts to increase circulation.

6. Finally open your chest (pointing your elbows backwards) three times.

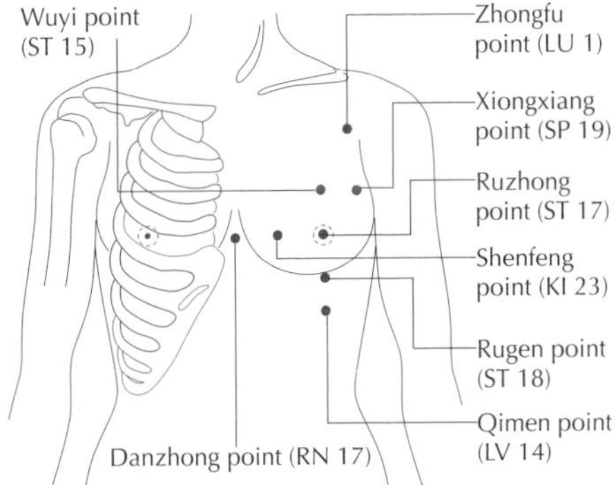

Fig. 49 Massaging the acupoints around the breast area are helpful.

2) Imbalance: Early Stage Breast Cysts

Breast cysts can occur as a result of menstrual irregularities, skipped menstrual cycles, too little blood flow during menstruation, or a combination of both. They are the result of accumulation of phlegm and liver qi stagnation.

The liver is responsible for regulating menstrual timing and a stagnated liver with accumulated mucus in the stomach meridian could cause worse PMS symptoms and cysts, according to TCM. Some of these symptoms can include, tender, sore, full, and painful breasts. In this condition, regulating liver qi and unblocking the phlegm may be useful.

Some tonics that help to prevent cysts also ensure that menstruation is both regular and that there is no stagnation of the blood. Ensuring that there is effective blood circulation of the uterus, and maintaining a smooth menstrual cycle can help to slow down the development of cysts.

Cysts that have a damp heat may grow and become large quite quickly. Whereas, cysts caused by stagnation without heat may grow at a slower pace. In this case, you would need to cool the condition using herbs or food remedies.

The following foods are recommended:

1. Taro is neutral, sweet, and spicy in properties and taste. Cooked taro can strengthen the spleen and stomach, and soften nodules and cysts. Boil the taro with beans, peas and carrots. When making mashed taro, add a little salt and pepper (adding spice helps to regulate qi), rosemary, cloves, coriander, natural butter, and olive oil. If you prefer to bake the taro, you could bake it in sesame oil or the fat from chicken stock. Chicken fat can be made by leaving chicken stock in the refrigerator overnight then scraping off the layer of fat on the top. Use this fat to bake the taro for a delicious and nutritious meal that can help to reduce the occurrence of breast cysts.

Taro Soup

Ingredients: taro 200 g, carrots 100 g, fresh or frozen peas 50 g

How to Prepare?

1. Peel the taro and carrots. Set aside the broad beans or dried green peas.
2. Place the taro and broad-beans into a pot. Add three pieces of ginger and some homemade chicken, beef or pork bone soup. Bring it to the boil then cook on a low heat for 35 minutes (if it is a large taro).
3. Add the carrots and peas. Bring to the boil again, then continue to cook for another ten minutes. Add salt, olive oil and chicken fat or sesame oil after cooking. Season with spices or pepper if you like.

2. Dandelion leaf is effective for cooling liver heat and tonifying the liver's blood. Dandelion, like artichoke, helps to combat deficiency of the liver. It also enters the meridians for the gallbladder, liver, and spleen so it is very good for all of these organs. It is very effective in regulating water retention in the liver meridian as water retention can be caused by liver heat, stagnation, or lack of liver yin.
3. Tangerine leaf is used very effectively for breast cysts. It is important to use leaves that have not been treated with any pesticides or chemicals. Simply take the leaves and dry them in the sun or a dehydrator. Use 12 g of dried leaf to make a tea. Boil the leaves in water for 20 minutes, then store this liquid in a container while you re-boil the leaves again in some fresh water for another twenty minutes. Once you have done so, add the two boiled portions of tea together and drink throughout the day.

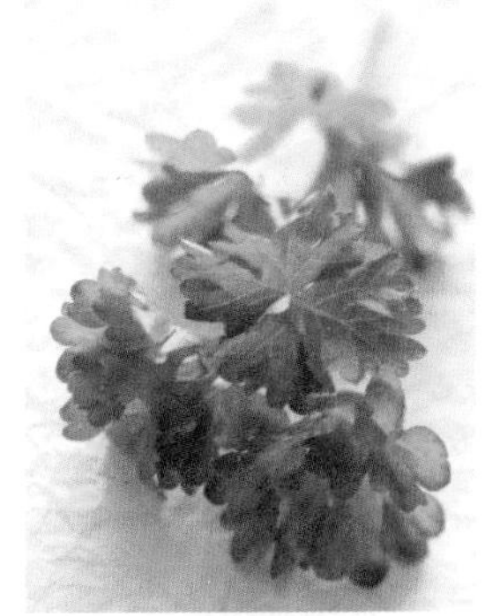

Fig. 50 Coriander

4. Coriander (fig. 50) is a fabulous

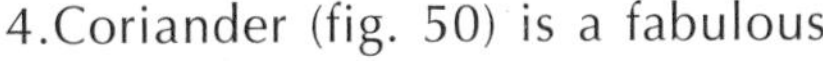

pungent and warm herb that can help to combat stagnation of qi and the accumulation of phlegm. Actually, all spices are effective in helping to remove stagnation and to combat dampness. This is due to the fact that they are arid and dry in nature. That is why people who live in areas in China with damper environments, include a lot more spices in their meals and are often known for their spicy food. Spices can also help to reduce excess body weight if added in small quantities to the diet.

3) Imbalance: Mastitis

Mastitis is a painful condition that can occur during breast-feeding, and can especially occur when feeding your first child. Your body system is weakened after giving birth for two to three weeks, according to Chinese medicine. Mastitis can occur when milk is not fully drained from the breast and an infection occurs. Symptoms can include local redness and swelling of the breast tissue, and fever.

Mastitis can occur when not pregnant, but this is far less common. Some people get mastitis once a year. This condition occurs as a result of a bacteria or virus and can also occur in the lung or throat, according to Western medicine. In TCM, the

Honeysuckle, Dried Mulberry Leaf, and Dandelion Leaf for Mastitis

Ingredients: dandelion 30 g, honeysuckle 12 g, dried mulberry leaf 12 g, 300 ml of water

How to Prepare?

1. Place the dandelion, honeysuckle, dried mulberry leaf and water in a pan.
2. Make a decoction by boiling the ingredients for 20 minutes, place the liquid aside. Add more water and re-boil the herbs again.
3. Add the two portions of liquid together and make sure all the herbs are strained out.
4. Drink it warm (20°C) twice a day for three days.

condition is caused by an accumulation of dampness and heat combining to trigger mastitis.

4) Imbalance: Breast Lumps (Solid Nodules)

A solid nodule occurs as a result of stagnation of qi that has turned to heat, according to Chinese medicine. It can also be caused by phlegm accumulation that has turned into blood stagnation. When someone has any of the above conditions, solid nodules are more likely to occur.

In this situation, you need to cool the heat and regulate blood circulation. Using this strategy can be effective for softening hard nodules. Solid nodules, tumors, or lumps also need to be prevented. They can occur in people who have qi deficiency and coldness, yin deficiency with hotness, or yang deficiency.

During pregnancy, a change in hormones prepares your breasts to produce breast milk, and your menstruation blood is no longer released. This blood stays inside the body and is absorbed to help provide extra nourishment for both the child and the mother. Breast-feeding can help to open up the meridians in the breast areas. If there are blockages in the breasts, breast-feeding may help unblock blockages for the breasts.

The following foods are recommended:

- Burdock seeds are often used in cancer treatments and are effective for removing phlegm and improving blood circulation. They are often taken to prevent solid nodules, or even used as a pre-cancer treatment once nodules have been surgically removed to stop them from coming back. Burdock seeds can be used to make a drink. You can pickle the root and eat it as an appetizer. If you are able to obtain the seeds, you might consider adding them to your breakfast.
- Lychee stones are very effective to dispel swelling. Dry

20 lychee stones in the sun or in a dehydrator, then grind them into powder. Use 9–12 g powder and add to water to make a decoction. It is very good for improving circulation, removing solid nodules, and eliminating pain.
- Other foods that are useful for softening nodules are seaweed, kelp, small red radish (eaten raw with different sauces), and lemon and lime juice added to hot water. It is important to use the meat and skin of the lime to achieve more effective results.

Flexible Tendons and Strong Nails

In order to improve the health of your tendons and nails, you might need to regulate liver qi and tonify the liver's blood or yin based on a diagnosis of excess or deficiency.

Excess is more common during middle age and for those who have a busy job or who regularly engage in buffet-style eating and banquets. Signs of excess include symptoms of fullness, pain, energy levels that are normal or excessive, extreme anger combined with hyperactivity, yellow urine, and constipation. In the case of the above symptoms, regulating and cooling the liver might be necessary.

Signs of deficiency include tenderness, fullness combined with dizzy spells, blurred vision, and exhaustion before or during menstruation. Symptoms can sometimes include dry mouth and feelings of thirst. This group would need to tonify the liver's blood and then seek to regulate liver qi.

Therefore, in order to make progress towards the attainment of better health, it is important to identify whether it is excess or weakness that is causing your symptoms. If the liver is not producing enough bile, then you need to facilitate bile production by choosing appropriate foods, relaxing, and not holding sustained feelings of anger. When you hold on to anger, you use up liver essence, which leads to liver weakness. In turn, you can be left feeling angrier, according to TCM thought.

1) Imbalance: Weakness of Tendons Breakage and Slow Nail Growth

Weak and soft tendons are usually a result of liver qi and blood deficiency.

The following foods are recommended:

- Asparagus is a very good food for both tonifying and regulating the liver. In particular, it can help to tonify the liver's yin (including body fluid and the liver's blood). It can also aid in reducing dampness and heat in the liver that can be caused as a result of heavy eating at banquets and the over consumption of oily foods.
- Fresh artichoke targets both the liver and gallbladder, and aids in the tonifying of the livers yin and blood. Furthermore, it helps to regulate the circulation of liver qi and facilitates the removal of liver qi stagnation.
- Warm and sweet in nature, pig or beef tendons have the function of strengthening the bones and tendons for weak people.
- Chicken feet are also good for the weak soft tendons due to their high collagen content.

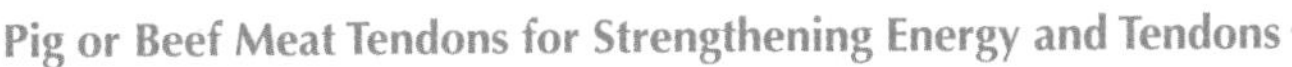

Pig or Beef Meat Tendons for Strengthening Energy and Tendons

Ingredients: pig or beef meat tendons 1000 g, water 3 liters, rice wine 120 ml, five spice 5 g, 1 bunch of spring onions, six pieces of ginger, soy sauce 200 ml

How to Prepare?

1. Clean all the ingredients thoroughly.
2. Add all the ingredients to a pot and bring to the boil. Continue to stew for 20 minutes.
3. Add all the ingredients into a slow cooker and stew it for another two hours.
4. Once cooked, slice the meat tendons into pieces, sprinkle with a tablespoon of beef juice.

2) Imbalance: Sprained Tendons

In China, the uncooked powder from the gardenia fruit is externally used for sprained muscles, tendons, and ligaments. It is cooling in nature and can reduce swelling.

A paste recipe for external use: 15 g of gardenia fruit powder, 5 g wheat flour and 10 ml water to make soft thin paste can be used to apply on the affected area.

3) Imbalance: Nail Fungus and Athlete's Foot

Athlete's foot and nail fungus have their root in a damp condition of the body. It is also a common condition that occurs as people age. Dampness might also be present on the nail, or made worse by wearing enclosed shoes all the time. Eating foods that promote dampness can also worsen it. Athlete's foot can be treated by soaking the feet in baking soda for 20 minutes for ten days.

External remedies for nail fungus:

- Thoroughly dry and ventilate shoes and feet. Sitting in the sun to dry the nail, this can further inhibit a nail fungus condition. There are also some useful natural remedies that can be used to treat nail fungus.
- Use fresh ginger or lime juice directly on the nail and leave for at least three minutes. Continue treatment until the fungus disappears. It will usually take at least two months.
- Soak the feet in the following concoction for ten days, and apply it to the surface of the nail: 20 g of stemona tuberosa lour (*bai bu*), with 12 g of rhubarb root (*da huang*), and 250 g of apple cider vinegar. Soak the herbs ten days before using. Please note that this is only for external use.

Healthy Color on the Skin

To remedy hyper-pigmentation, it might be a good idea to clear the stagnation in the blood. To even the skin tone when white spots are present, it may be necessary to tonify the blood.

1) Imbalance: Pigmentation after Giving Birth

After a woman has given birth, she might bear body fluid and blood weakness. She can seek to regulate her liver and hormones with certain food, herb, acupressure, and massage therapies. Natural fruit acids (such as a lemon juice mask on the skin) may also help to lessen pigmentation.

When women are pregnant, more liver blood is distributed to the growing baby. Consequently, the quantity of blood to the surface of the mother's skin and face are lessened so she may develop some pigmentation. Strengthening liver yin and blood during pregnancy can help to limit this condition.

The following foods are recommended:

- Artichoke is sweet, bitter, and salty in taste. It is cool in energy, acting on the nourishing and moistening the dryness. At same time, it speeds up energy movement, regulates heat, and reduces water retention.
- Beetroot is sweet in taste, neutral in energy, acting on the channels of the liver and heart, and tonifying the blood. This is helpful for people with anemia. The vitamin C in beetroot is good to remove pigmentation.
- Spinach is sweet in taste, cool in energy, acting on the channels of the liver, small and large intestines and stomach. Spinach strengthens the five *zang*-viscera, descending abnormally ascending qi, regulating the middle-energize, clearing heat, nourishing the blood to reduce pigmentation, arresting bleeding, keeping the fluid in body, moistening dryness, tonifying the liver, and brightening the eyes.
- 100% pearl powder has been famously used in China for pigmentation, especially after pregnancy. It can help to regulate the central nervous system, leading to better sleep and reducing the pigmentation that results from lack of sleep. It is good for blood circulation and brightens the complexion. It is also for exteral use. It can easily be absorbed into the

skin, and helps to open blockages and reduce color. It is also useful against shingles as it helps to cool the skin, supports the nervous system, and combats scarring. Mix the powder with vitamin E and apply to the affected area.

2) Imbalance: White Spots and Vitiligo

External remedies:

- Fig tonic (fig. 51). Slice 250 g of fig (fruit and leaves) and soak in 50% alcohol for seven days. Apply the solution on the affected area twice a day for two weeks.

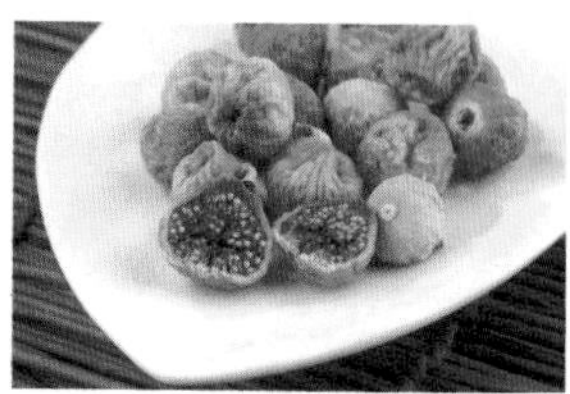

Fig. 51 Dried fig

- Gardenia fruit infusion. Soak 25 g of gardenia, 25 g Fructus Psoraleae (*bug gu zhi*) to 200 ml of 75% alcohol for seven days. Then apply the infusion on the affected area, twice a day. Continue for two weeks.

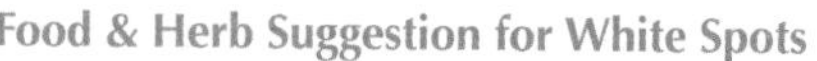

Food & Herb Suggestion for White Spots

TCM doctors often prescribe the following herbal and super-food mixture for tonifying the blood in order to prevent and cure white spots on the skin. The ingredients can be bought from a TCM pharmacy, but it is recommended that you work with your own TCM doctor to ensure the tonic is appropriate for your own individual constitution.

Materials: raw fo-ti root (*sheng shou wu*) 2 g; Chinese angelica root 2 g; safflower 1 g; peach kernel 1 g; Fructus Tribuli 3 g; jujube 2 g; root of common wild peony (radix paeoniae rubra, *chi shao*) 1 g; wolfberry 2 g; 100 ml of water

How to Prepare?

1. Ground all the materials into powder.
2. Option 1: Mix all the powder with 100 ml of hot water and stir well. Divide into two portions. Drink one portion in the morning after breakfast and the other portion after dinner.

   Option 2: Mix all the powder with half a tablespoon of honey and eat with whole grain bread or crackers.
3. This recipe should be taken for three weeks.

3) Imbalance: Dark Pigmentation, Purple Dots on the Tongue Company with Dull Ache in the Rib Area

The recipes provided below could help to clear liver blood stagnation and can aid in the removal of skin pigmentation. Detoxifying your liver can help reduce and prevent the build-up of pigmentation.

The following foods are recommended:

- Saffron is neutral and can be used for a hot or cold constitution, suitable for anyone. You may use 0.5–1 g of saffron to make a tea. Boil water and pour it into your cup with the saffron inside. Cover with a lid for five minutes. Drink two times each day and make sure you eat the flowers afterwards.
- Safflower is a cheaper version of saffron. It has a warm spicy taste, and should be used with caution by those who have a hot/yang constitution, thin blood, and trouble with blood clotting. You should use 3 g of safflower and prepare using the same method as above.
- Peach kernel (*tao ren*) is a powerful remedy against pigmentation caused by blood stagnation. Prepare the peach kernel by drying some peach seeds in the sun or in a dehydrator. Once dried, cook it in a frying pan (without oil) until it turns yellow. You can add some sea salt. Either grind it into a fine powder or crush it into small pieces. You can eat 6–9 g, begin with 6 g and work your way up to 9 g. Alternatively, you can add it to bread or pancakes. Don't eat too much of it as it contains a lot of oil. If you get diarrhea, then stop taking it and chose a more gentle anti-stagnation remedy. Those who have loose stools or excessive bleeding should not use it. Likewise, those who have a blood deficiency or who bleed easily should choose another remedy.
- Chinese angelica root is a wonderful herb that fights

pigmentation and helps to nourish the blood. You can make a nourishing chicken or lamb soup with it. If you were using 250 g of meat and 1 L of water, add 9–12 g of Chinese angelica root. You can use a small cotton bag to place the herbs in and remove it once the soup is fully cooked. You can buy premade Chinese angelica root tablets if you prefer. Chinese angelica root is a warming herb and should not be used with those who have a yin deficiency (hot constitution), damp heat, or excessive fire condition.

External remedies for pigmentation:

- Using dried and powdered persimmon leaf can counteract pigmentation. Once you have ground it into a powder, add it to some olive oil and lemon juice, and make a paste to apply locally on the pigmentation.

Don't Let Anger Build Up

It is very important to express yourself and avoid suppressing or bottling up your emotions, according to TCM. Finding positive strategies to move from the past situations that make you feel angry is vital. It can smooth and balance liver qi, and avoid liver stagnation and hyperactivity. There are manual strategies you could use to support the liver and to help reduce excess anger.

- Smiling. It will tone the muscles that pull upwards and will also help you produce "happy chemicals" such as endorphins, oxytocin, serotonin, and dopamine. These happy chemicals can also aid your body in detoxification, make you to feel a greater sense of wellbeing, help you sleep better, and can affect your endocrine system.
- Self-massage. Use the palm and heel of your hand to massage just below the ribs where the liver is situated and liver meridian passes through (fig. 52). Massage up and down along the front of the ribs, following the natural

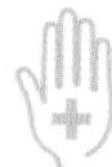

Self-Massage to Regulate the Liver Qi

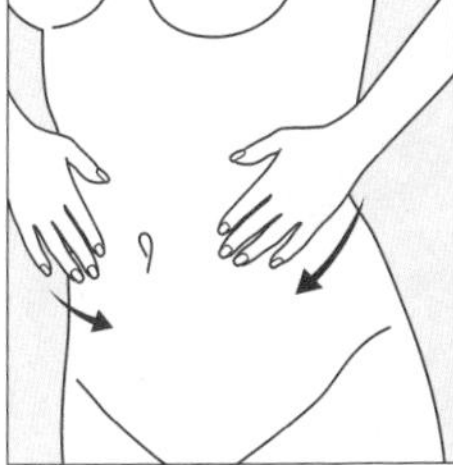

Fig. 52 Massage from the side of breast along the front of the ribs down following the natural curves, repeat for 20 times.

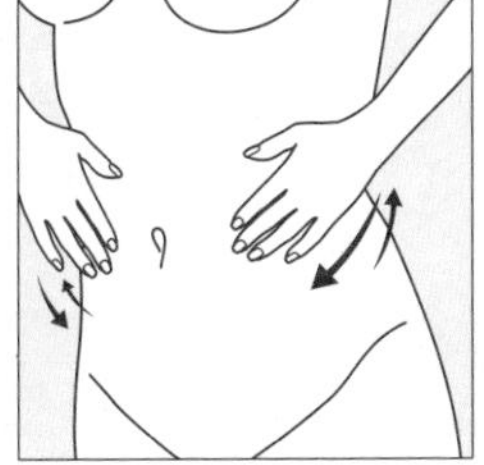

Fig. 53 Massage upward and downward from the side of breast along the front of the ribs down to the belly, repeat 20 times.

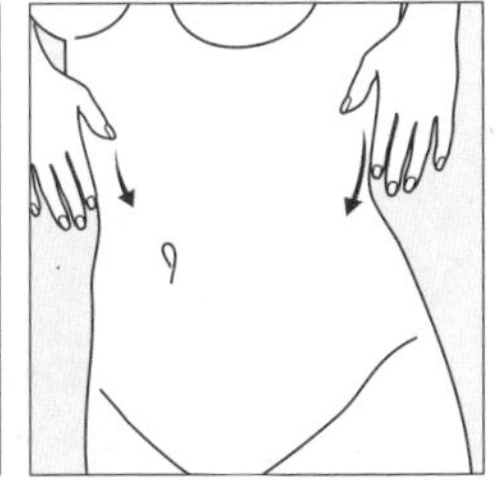

Fig. 54 Massage from the armpit below straight downwards to the waist bone, repeat for 20 times.

curves 20–30 times (fig. 53). Self-massage can stimulate liver qi and blood movements. Some people with liver qi stagnation may become tearful and the qi and blood begins to move again (fig. 54).

- Watch a sad movie. When the liver is stressed, you might find yourself regularly on the verge of tears. Watching a sad movie that makes you cry can assist the removal of liver stagnation and help the liver rebalance. Once the stagnation is released, then the energy in the liver can flow smoothly again.

Your incredible and hard-working liver works tirelessly day and night to keep you healthy and it rarely complains. Making minor changes can have powerful affects on this amazing organ and can ensure that your eyes and nails sparkle. Looking after your liver can help to balance your emotions, reducing feelings of anger and anxiety. Beautiful breasts and blemish free skin can also be attributed to a healthy liver system. Next up is the spleen.

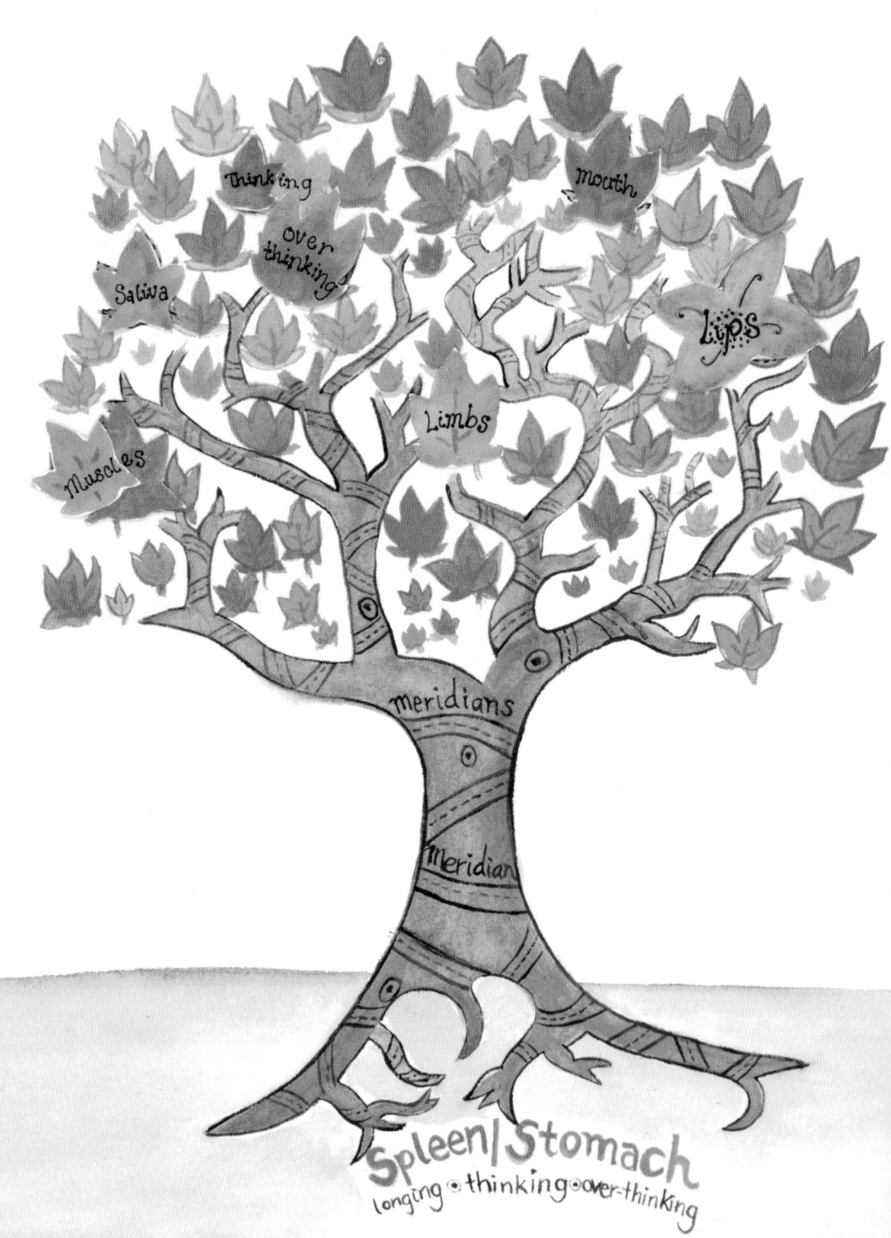
Thinking
mouth
over thinking
Saliva
Lips
Limbs
Muscles
meridians
Meridian
Spleen|Stomach
longing thinking over-thinking

CHAPTER SEVEN

The Spleen System

Roots

- *Zang*-organ: the TCM concept of "spleen". It refers to the organs with digestive functions including the spleen, pancreas, and part of small intestine.
- *Fu*-organ: stomach
- Emotion of longing and thinking

Trunk and Branches

- Meridians: Taiyin Spleen Meridian of Foot, Yangming Stomach Meridian of Foot

Leaves

- Fresh breath in mouth
- Thin saliva when eating from parotid gland to help digestion
- Firm and elastic muscles
- Flexible limbs

Fruits

- Emotion of longing and desire (also part of the "roots" system)
- Mood of thinking or over-thinking (also part of the "roots" system)

Flowers

- Rosy, nourished and smooth lips

Left Fig. 55 The liver system tree

1. Basic Facts about the Spleen System

When we refer to the "spleen" in TCM, we are not only referring to the spleen organ, but other organs with digestive functions, such as the spleen, pancreas and part of the small intestine. The spleen meridians, related emotions, lips, muscles, and limbs are also included in this system.

As mentioned earlier, every organ is paired with another organ. In this case, the spleen is paired with the stomach. In this special relationship, the spleen is the *zang*-organ and the stomach is the *fu*-organ.

The meridians of this system are the Taiyin Spleen Meridian of Foot and Yangming Stomach Meridian of Foot.

There is an old Chinese saying, "The spleen opens into the mouth, and you can tell how healthy your spleen system is through your taste in mouth and saliva." This is still true, as many TCM practitioners still observe the mouth and saliva during their clinical assessment if the patient is describing symptoms of a spleen imbalance.

The emotion of longing (desire) and the mood of thinking or over-thinking are the fruits of this tree, but they are also part of the root system.

The flowers of the spleen tree are the lips.

2. Functions of the Spleen

The spleen has several main functions, according to TCM.

Firstly, once you begin to consume foods and liquids, the spleen system begins to digest them. A healthy spleen system will effectively separate nutrition from waste and will help you absorb the nutrients you need. We call this process "transformation".

Secondly, the spleen system helps to produce qi, blood, and

body fluids from the nutrition you have absorbed, and brings them up to the lung and head. From there, qi, blood, and body fluids are distributed to nourish the whole body. These life giving substances promote the healthy functions of the all the organs. We call this process "transportation".

The third function is called "governing the blood flow within the vessel". In TCM, the spleen plays an important role in the prevention of bleeding and strengthens the texture of the blood veins.

"Transformation": Separating Nutrition and Waste

"You are what you eat" was a popular saying in the 1990's, though this is only partially true. "You are what you absorb" is a better expression. And what you absorb is dependent upon how healthy your spleen system is.

Once you consume food and liquid, the stomach and spleen begin to digest it. These organ systems are responsible for the rhythm of the stomach known as "peristaltic contractions". The spleen also plays a role in producing digestive acid, which is vital for the effective break down of the food. Those with too little stomach acid will inevitably suffer from digestive troubles.

As mentioned earlier, part of the small intestine is included in the spleen system. It is in the small intestine where nutrition is separated from waste, and vitamins and minerals are absorbed effectively. Any remaining waste will be pushed into the colon.

Every cell in your body needs nourishment. The effectiveness of the spleen system will dictate how much nutrition your cells receive from the food and drink you consume. If your spleen energy is low, you might lack digestive-fire, and may not be able to absorb all the nutrients you should. However, supporting the spleen system can help your body rebalance digestive issues.

"Transportation": Ascending the "Clear"

In TCM, the nutrients you absorb from your diet are transformed into qi, blood, and body fluids. The term "ascending the clear" refers to the process whereby qi ascends up to the head and lung. We must remember that wherever qi goes, blood and body fluids follow, so as qi rises up to the head and lung, so does your nourishing blood and body fluids. With the help of the lung, qi, blood, and body fluids are then distributed to the entire body, which nourishes every cell with their life-giving properties. The term "clear" refers to the qi, blood, and body fluids that ascend. For the purpose of this chapter, we will refer to these three important substances as "clear qi".

Qi, blood, and body fluids are vital for the whole body. And, the spleen system is the first organ system that begins the transportation process.

About 20% to 30% of your "clear qi" is sent upward directly to your head. As a result, your eyes, nose, and ears function optimally. If you regularly feel muddy headed, it may be because your spleen is not performing its function of providing nourishment to your head. Being forgetful or getting dizzy often can originate from a weak spleen system.

About 70% to 80% of your "clear qi" is sent upward to the lung. From there, with the help of your breathing, nutrition is distributed to the whole body.

The function of "ascending the clear" also plays a vital role in stabilizing the internal organs in their original location and not allowing them to collapse. You may have heard of stomach, kidney, uterus, and anal prolapses. When spleen qi is low, it is unable to perform the role of "ascending the clear", resulting in an increased risk of organ prolapses.

"Transportation": Descending the Waste

The spleen system also directs the transportation of the waste (solid and water) downward to the colon in order to let it come out through the lower orifices.

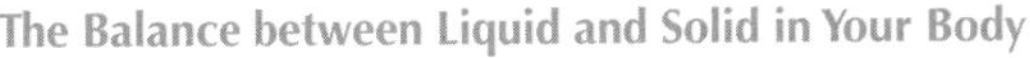

The Balance between Liquid and Solid in Your Body

As we know, fluids can travel in and out of the veins to nourish body tissues and cells. When there is not enough fluid in the veins, the blood can become sticky and sluggish due to an imbalance between the liquid and solid elements in your blood.

So it is important to have a normal amount of body fluids in you system. You may have heard that your body is approximately 70% water and this is very important because your body fluids help to carry qi and oxygen, and ensure healthy blood and smooth flowing lymph. Adequate circulation of liquid is important for a balanced metabolism.

Jin ye is an important concept of Chinese culture, "jin" means pure water and "ye" means nourished liquid. Chinese people do not drink a lot of pure water. They prefer nourishing soups and teas because there are plenty of nutrients inside of liquid. Popular soup ingredients include bones, root vegetables, fish, sea-plants (such as kelp, marine algae, seaweed), and sea salt (or well salt in inland regions).

Water retention and oedema can be caused by spleen imbalances, particularly in the legs and below the midsection (from the belly button down). Even if you are able to excrete a good amount of urine daily, you may still suffer with edema in the ankles and legs due to the fact that your spleen is not transporting and circulating your body fluids adequately.

Governing the Blood Flow within the Vessels

Blood needs both "holding power" and "promoting power" to ensure it goes in the right directions. "Promoting power" ensures that your blood circulates smoothly, and "holding power" ensures that you do not bleed excessively in the event of an accident.

The spleen has "holding power", which can be likened to blood coagulation and the effective functioning of platelets, according to TCM.

If there is a spleen weakness, blood-clotting mechanisms may

Dampness and Your Spleen

The spleen likes dryer environments rather than damper ones. This is because the spleen is susceptible to an "invasion of dampness". If dampness invades the spleen, then its function of "ascending the clear", holding the blood, and its role in transportation and transformation will be affected.

Dampness can affect spleen function as a result of eating too many sweet foods, dairy and oily foods or living in a damp environment with high humidity.

Damp geological environments with high humidity affect the spleen. Humidity can be absorbed through the skin and feelings of heaviness, a muddy head, a sticky mouth, and the inability to keep your eyes open may result. Furthermore, oily skin, sluggish limbs, and incomplete stool evacuation may occur. Many people experience these symptoms when humidity is high.

Too many dairy foods, sugar, and deep fried foods can cause dampness in the body. Those who have issues with their pancreas and intolerance to sugar might find that the source of their problems are coming from the spleen. They might be more likely to experience fluid retention and even edema.

The following foods are recommended for expelling the dampness:

- Drink tea. Green and Oolong tea is recommended. If you have a cold constitution, then you can drink black tea, without milk and sugar. Milk and sugar will negate the positive effects of drinking tea in the first place.
- Take something bitter, such as bitter melon (fig. 56), chamomile, or feverfew (which is similar to chrysanthemum).
- Those who identify themselves as having a spleen deficiency or weakness should not indulge in too many sweet foods. For instance, two pieces of chocolate will not cause dampness, but a whole block in one sitting might.

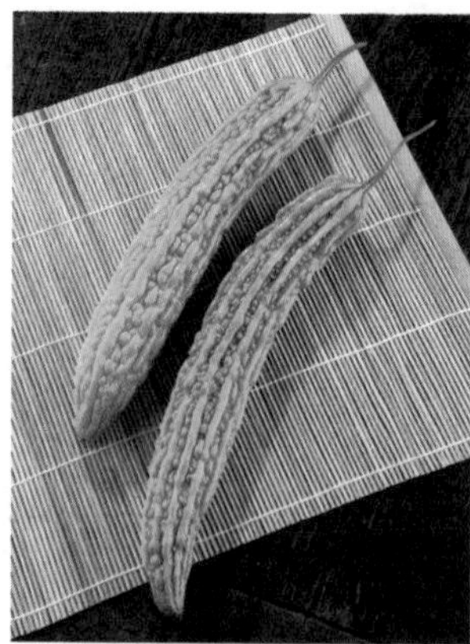

Fig. 56 Bitter melons

not work very well, causing an individual to bruise more easily. If you find yourself getting a lot of bruises after massage, then you may need to tonify the spleen system.

Another function of the spleen is to prevent extra bleeding. Some people have a lot of uterus bleeding outside their set menstrual period and perhaps also experience bruises that occur easily below the waist area.

Symptoms of exhaustion, unusual bleeding, diarrhea, and bloating in the stomach and abdominal area are other signs of a spleen imbalance. These symptoms can be addressed by treating the spleen system.

3. Meridians of the Spleen System

The Taiyin Spleen Meridian of Foot begins from the inside edge of the big toe and travels across the arch of the foot, over the front of the ankle up inside the leg all the way up to the groin. It then passes over the groin and up the waistline, moving towards the spleen and stomach (fig. 57). This meridian goes up both sides of the oesophagus into the throat area where it attaches to the roof of the tongue and travels under the tongue.

The Yangming Stomach Meridian of Foot starts from the side of the nose, travels up the outer edges of each side of the nose bridge, and then goes under the eye to the middle of the cheek. It then crosses below the nose and moves around the corner of the mouth, lips, and to both sides of the middle of the chin. It then moves up the jaw line and splits into two paths. One path travels up the jaw, past the ear, and up to the corner of the hairline (fig. 58).

The second path travels from the edge of the jawbone down to the front of the neck, where it goes to the chest area, through the diaphragm and then enters the stomach and the spleen. The

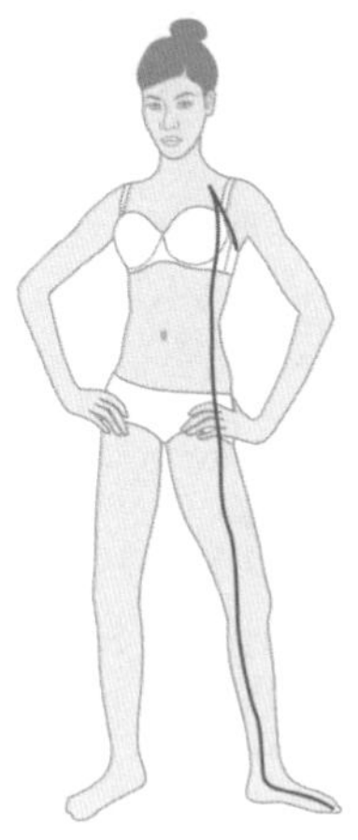

Fig. 57 Taiyin Spleen Meridian of Foot

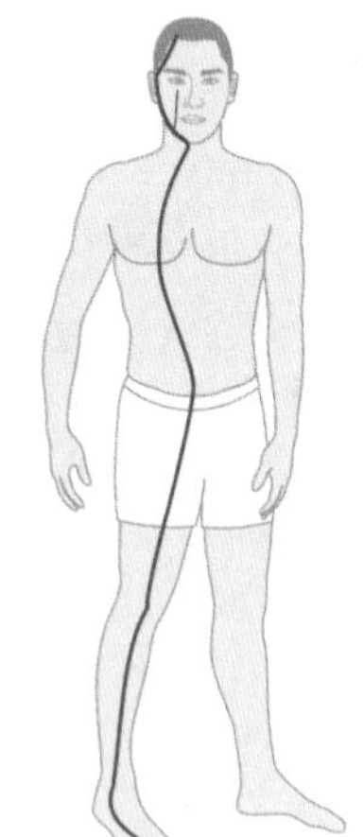

Fig. 58 Yangming Stomach Meridian of Foot

superficial channel travels down to the breast and abdomen, and then moves down the front of the leg across the knee down the front of the lower leg on top of the middle of the foot, and ends at the side of the second toe.

4. Spleen System and Beauty

Your spleen determines whether you have a strong or weak constitution. You are born with a congenital constitution, but you are responsible for your acquired constitution and looking after your spleen system is vital for this.

When the spleen system is functioning normally, spleen qi should go up and stomach qi should go down. If spleen qi becomes stuck in the mid-section, it may affect the normal movement patterns of the spleen system. Since your spleen assists in the production and transportation of qi and blood, it also plays a role in growth and development.

Symptoms of exhaustion, unusual bleeding, diarrhea, bloating in the stomach and abdominal area, poor appetite, dizzy spells, and becoming forgetful can all be signs that your spleen system is out of balance.

These symptoms can be addressed by treating the spleen system. When treating the spleen, it may be necessary to also support your heart system as the heart system can help to regulate the spleen's emotions.

Mouth: the "Opening" of the Spleen

Bing cong kou ru is an important saying in Chinese culture, it means disease comes in or enters into the body through the mouth. This concepts pertains to the idea that what you ingest can bring health or harm to your body. Of course, this saying also takes into consideration that viruses and bacteria can enter through your mouth. But even more important is that you can prevent disease and influence your health by what you choose to put into your mouth.

Food selection is an important point of discussion in Chinese culture. There are three central ideas that are pertinent for this topic.

First, make good food choices. Selecting a wide range of healthy, unprocessed foods in their natural state. It is also a good idea to choose local, organic, and non-GMO foods that are in season. Eating until you are 70% full is a good habit.

Second, selecting food based on your individual constitution. The concept of bio-individuality is not a new notion in China. The saying, "one man's food is another man's poison" has been at the heart of food choices for generations. Choosing food according to the type of "stomach" you have has always been an aim for those wishing to maintain good health.

The different stomach types include: damp, cold, warm, acid, and a stomach that lacks enough acid. Food choices that suit your constitution can help to ensure you effectively absorb the foods you eat. For instance, someone with a cold stomach would not do well eating a lot of cold or cooling foods. Doing so may impair their ability to absorb the nutrients from those specific meals and may also injure the spleen system as a whole. Some lucky individuals have a relatively balanced stomach and do not need to pay a lot of attention when selecting foods accordingly.

When you consume foods you should pay attention to the reaction in your body afterwards. If you have no negative symptoms such as bloating, hiccups, diarrhea, or gas, then the food you have eaten may have been a good choice for your body.

You can further support your "stomach type" and constitution by adding food remedies. For instance, if you have less acidity in your stomach, you might add more vinegar, and sweet and sour food to your diet. If you have too much acidity, you might avoid foods that are too acidic.

It is also important to consider how your body is structured based on your ancestry and current health status. For instance, someone who has had their gallbladder removed through surgery may need to make different food choices than someone who hasn't.

What your ancestors ate can also dictate which foods might be more suited to your individual constitution, as our bodies do evolve based on our ancestry. If your ancestors lived by the ocean, you might easily digest a lot of seafood. If your ancestors ate a lot of meat, your small intestine might be slightly shorter than someone whose ancestors ate a lot of vegetables. We are all different in our constitutional makeup so why should we all eat the same food? It would be impossible to eat all the different types of foods in the world so it only makes sense to absorb a wide variety of nutrients based on locally grown foods that align with our constitutional typing.

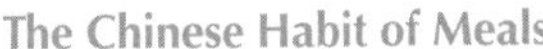

The Chinese Habit of Meals

Meals in China usually consist of several vegetable dishes, a small amount of meat, a small bowl of rice or noodles, and a soup.

Organ meats are included in the diet and all parts of the animal are valued. Meat is more of an accompaniment and is usually cooked with another type of vegetable such as bamboo fungus or lily bulb for instance, adding to the overall quantity of vegetables in a meal.

Sugar is kept to a minimum and is sometimes added to meals, but only in small amounts. Natural sources of sugar such as jujube and wolfberries are often included in the diet. Desserts in China are usually not that sweet.

There are also many types of herbal foods with anti-aging properties that are regularly consumed according to the constitution of the individual.

It has been discovered that Chinese people tend to have slightly longer small intestines than Western people. This has occurred as a result of thousands of years of cultural dietary choices.

Third, choosing healthy food that your body can absorb. Absorption is affected by the quality of the food you consume and your spleen's ability to transform and transport it. The Chinese prefer foods that are more easily digested.

For instance, even though it is well-known that brown rice contains more B-vitamins than white rice, Chinese people have long known that brown rice is more difficult to digest. For this reason, they have always paid attention to its preparation with methods such as soaking and grinding. Both of these methods help to make brown rice more digestible. Many Chinese families will soak brown rice for five hours before using it, or may use a device to crush it. Then they would cook it together with white rice in order to further enhance the digestion process.

Saliva: Helping Digestion

Saliva from the parotid gland that is produced when you see or smell food belongs to the spleen system in TCM. It helps you to swallow and digest your food. It also helps to moisten the mouth.

You should have sufficient saliva, but not so much that you are constantly dribbling. Unless you are a teething toddler, then some dribbling is acceptable, of course.

People who dribble a lot when sleeping or talking may have spleen issues that are in need of resolution. A mouth that is too dry (despite having consumed enough water) may be an indication that your spleen system is not efficiently sending body fluids to the mouth.

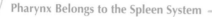

Pharynx Belongs to the Spleen System

The Pharynx is the passage way leading down from the mouth and nose to the oesophagus. It belongs to the spleen system in Chinese medicine.

The spleen and stomach meridians both pass over the pharynx and it relies on these organ systems to be healthy. Problems with the pharynx may be addressed by treating stomach function.

Lips: Flower of the Spleen

Traditional Chinese medicine looks at the color and texture of the lips as an indication of the TCM spleen health. The color and moistness of your lips depend on normal circulation of qi and blood. Since the spleen is one of the primary producers of qi and blood, the beauty and health of your lips are reliant upon this very important organ system. Normal lips should be pink or dark red in color, depending on your nationality. They should be moist, and not dry or cracked. Peeling skin and frequent cracks in the corners of the mouth can be linked to a decline in spleen function.

Furthermore, a healthy spleen can help provide some protection against the herpes virus and also reduce the occurrence of outbreaks.

A strong spleen will facilitate the proper transformation and transportation of the food and drink you ingest and ensure that qi, blood, and body fluids are able to make their way to your lips.

Luscious lips are a result of your spleen's ability to perform its function of "ascending the clear".

Issues relating to the lips might be linked back to the spleen system.

- Muscle shrinkage around the lips can be related to spleen function. Looking after this organ system can prevent atrophy and the sagging of the muscles around the lips.
- Pale lips may indicate spleen qi and blood deficiency.
- Dry and cracked lips may indicate that qi and body fluids are not ascending properly.

Please note that purple colored lips and cheeks are more related to heart function or blockages in the blood vessels and would be treated by addressing the heart system.

Muscles: Tissue of the Spleen

In traditional Chinese medicine, the muscles include the fat, fascia, and the muscles themselves. The muscles, fat, and fascia along with the skin, provide a protective barrier against invading factors. They also protect our internal organs and hold them in the right places. They accompany the ligaments, tendons, bones, and joints to help us move.

Healthy spleen function will create strong, well-developed muscles. All the muscles in our body depend on nutrition produced by the spleen system to grow strong and to remain firm. It will also help to prevent water retention and cellulite.

Some people in puberty who are experiencing digestive issues might find that their muscle growth is very slow. Your muscle's growth depends on the spleen's ability to absorb nutrients. If you are having trouble developing muscle, investigating spleen function from a TCM perspective might offer some helpful solutions.

Some people have small muscles, but their muscles are strong. These people may or may not be a fan or exercise,

However, they can thank a healthy spleen system for their muscle integrity. Other people might find that even though their muscles are big, they are soft and lack strength. As mentioned earlier, firm muscles depend on sufficient qi and blood, which is made in the spleen system and distributed by it.

Addressing spleen function first may treat muscle atrophy, lack of muscle strength and even some cases of paralysis. Other organ systems may also need attention. For instance, paralysis of an arm as a result of a stroke. In this case, both the spleen and heart system might be addressed.

Some people experience a lot of muscle atrophy and sagging at a young age. Muscle atrophy and sagging shouldn't be extreme before the age of 70. If the spleen is weak, it cannot support muscle function and its holding ability. Then muscle sagging can occur.

Some women may find that they begin to develop this condition after menopause as a result of changing hormones. A TCM doctor might treat the spleen to rectify this condition. In China, doctors may treat muscle atrophy that has occurred as a result of an accident by strengthening the spleen system before administering other treatments such as rehabilitation exercises.

Limbs: Outer Territory of the Spleen

In addition to the muscles, the spleen also impacts the four limbs. It helps the muscles in the limbs remain firm, coordinated, and strong. Likewise, exercises that involve the four limbs can help digestive system function.

Thinking and Longing: Emotion of the Spleen

In Chinese medicine, the spleen's emotions are longing and thinking, or overthinking.

Longing can be a natural part of life. For instance, a teenager might long to develop friendships with the opposite sex, or someone might long to see an old friend. There is also a longing that can occur for chocolate or coffee.

Likewise, thinking is also a normal part of life. We need to think and make decisions on a daily basis. We might need to carefully plan a trip or schedule in advance. We also may need to absorb knowledge when we study or begin a new job. These are all normal processes within daily life and a healthy spleen function will be able to support these activities.

It is only when longing becomes excessive and out of control, or someone begins to overthink everything to the point where it affects their appetite and eating patterns that these functions become damaging to the spleen system.

TCM believes that excessive thinking and longing can disturb the movements of spleen qi and cause qi to become blocked. So it is important to endeavor not to overthink or let our longings get out of control. When going through periods of stress, change, decision-making, or difficult study, it is a good idea to support the spleen system.

Work-a-holics tend to scoff their food while they continue to work without taking a break. This is not healthy for the spleen system as thinking consumes up a lot of spleen qi that you should be using to digest your food at meal times.

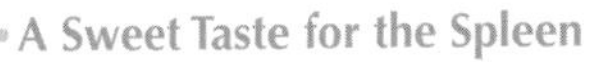

The spleen controls thinking. For those working hard or studying, a strong spleen system will be advantageous. The sweet taste affects the spleen, according to TCM.

In times of stress, a little sweetness in your diet can help to support and strengthen the spleen and stomach.

Please note that sweet food needs to be eaten in moderation and in a reasonable quantity. Too many sweets with dairy (for instance, dairy and sugar) is not great for your body or your spleen. It can add to the accumulation of phlegm and may contribute towards a damp condition in your body.

5. Beauty Problems and Enhancement

Now we will discuss the beauty concerns that are related to your spleen system and will provide some food options and herbal recipes that will benefit your spleen.

We will include some remedies for common beauty issues such as edema, cellulite, saggy skin, weight issues, bloating, bad breath, under-eye bags, and how to maintain beautiful lips.

Staying Fit

Maintaining a normal range of body weight, a relative balance between body fat and muscles, and a solid and lasting physique are important to us.

1) Imbalance: Water Retention and Edema

Those who have issues with their pancreas and intolerance to sugar might find that the source of their problems are coming from the spleen. They might be more likely to experience water retention and even edema.

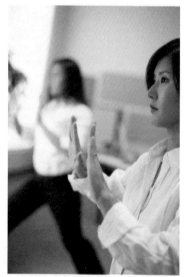

Fig. 59 Exercise is vital for the health of spleen.

Water retention is less severe than edema (which creates more swelling). Some people may find that they get very swollen legs after flying for ten hours or more. This is a sign of spleen weakness that has left someone more susceptible to accumulating dampness in your body. Water retention is often caused by the spleen's inability to effectively transform and transport the fluids

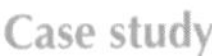

Case study

Symptoms: Every year between spring and summer, Sarah, a 38-year-old female, suffered from ankle swelling for several months. Like clockwork, every year at the same time, her ankles would swell up during these seasons. Whenever she had to fly, her entire legs would swell up to her knees. The swelling would improve in the mornings and become worse in the afternoons and evenings. When she pressed her ankle, deep impressions would linger for a few seconds. Sometimes her face would become puffy. Her body always felt heavy and lethargic. Her tongue had a thick white coating in the middle and she had teeth marks along the edges of her tongue.

Analysis: During spring and summer, there is a transition time when the environment is very damp, according to TCM. Some people are more susceptible to dampness invading the spleen at these times. The meridian of the spleen runs along the inside of the ankle and calf and those who are susceptible may experience more swelling along this meridian. The teeth marks along the edge of the tongue further indicate spleen weakness and are caused by the tongue swelling.

Treatment: Strengthening and warming the spleen can effectively treat this condition. It is also important to remove dampness and increase urine output. Herbs and functional foods are very good for this purpose. In Sarah's case, she consumed winter melon (*dong gua*) soup for a few weeks and the water retention was gone after 16 dosages. The following year, she began the treatment just before the damp season arrived and she remained symptom free.

in your body.

People with a weak spleen system might feel very sensitive to humidity in comparison to those with a strong one.

Exercise is vital for the spleen as it moves all of your muscles, and since the spleen governs your muscles, your regular workout can also tone and exercise your spleen. Additionally, moving your four limbs is particularly beneficial to the spleen (fig. 59).

In order to treat water retention and edema, it is important to treat dampness, strengthen the spleen organ, try not to overthink things, and pay attention to your food choices.

The following foods are recommended:

- Corn silk (the string found around the corn beneath the leaves) can be made into a soup to counteract dampness (fig. 60).

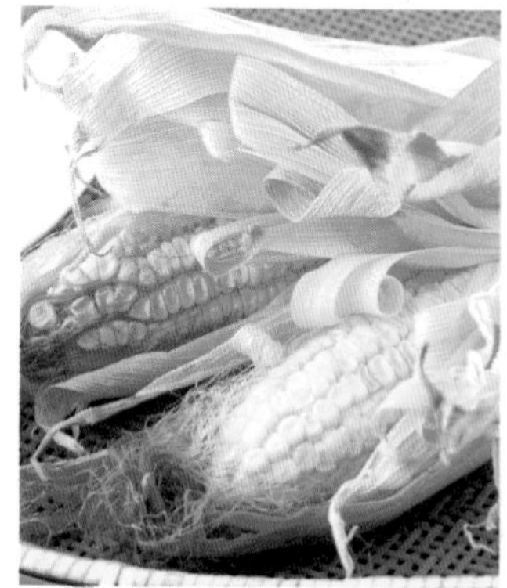

Fig. 60 Corn silk can be made into tea.

- Sichuan pepper is warming to the middle *jiao* and is effective in dispersing cold, expelling dampness, and reducing pain. It can stop abdominal pain accompanied by vomiting and diarrhea. Furthermore, it can help reduce feelings of coldness in the joints as well as swelling and pain.
- Pearl barley can help eliminate water retention through the urine. Simultaneously, it can help the spleen to improve its own functions of water metabolism. In China, pearl barley is regularly consumed as a soup or porridge.
- Tea, especially green tea, is a diuretic. It helps to increase urination, relieve edema, and treat phlegm, and bad breath. Conditions commonly found in smokers such as daily morning phlegm, mucus, and persistent bronchitis are known as damp conditions and drinking green tea can help provide some relief. Chewing on the brewed tea leaves can also help to mask bad breath.
- The seeds, skin, and fibrous part that holds the seeds of winter melon are the most functional part of winter melon.

The following recipes are mainly for seasonal edema. When using these remedies, it is important to ensure you do not have a heart, liver, or kidney disease causing the edema. For these conditions, you need to be under the supervision of your doctor.

Winter Melon Soup with Kelp

Ingredients: winter melon 500 g, rehydrate kelp 100 g, water 2 L (serve four person)

How to Prepare?

1. Wash the winter melon and cut into rectangles about 1 cm thick. Include some seeds, string and skin (if organic).
2. Put the skin, seeds, and fiber into a cotton bag.
3. Add a little oil in a pan and stir-fry the winter melon for two minutes.
4. Add the winter melon, cotton bag and kelp into a pot with boiling water, and bring to the boil.
5. Turn the heat down and cook for 20 minutes. Add salt, pepper (Sichuan pepper if you have some) to garnish.

Azuki Bean Soup

Ingredients: azuki beans 30 g, water 300 ml (This is a day supply, you can prepare three days' supply at once)

How to Prepare?

1. Wash the beans and drain the water.
2. Soak 30 g of azuki beans overnight.
3. Put soaked azuki beans and water to a pot. Bring to the boil for 5 minutes.
4. Add the soup to a slow cooker. Cook for 1.5 hours. If you don't have a slow cooker you could cook it in a pot on a low heat.
5. Add salt, jujubes, or honey to taste. You could also add some gingko nuts, lotus seeds and serve it as a dessert.
6. Drink the soup and eat the beans.

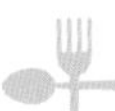

Pearl Barley Porridge

Ingredients: 60 g of pearl barley, 30 g of rice, 600 ml of water

How to Prepare?

1. Soaked the pearl barley for at least 30 minutes.
2. Mix the pearl barley, rice, and water together. Cook in a rice cooker or pressure cooker for 30 minutes.
3. Use two to three times each week to reduce water retention.

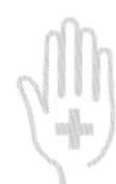

Other Remedy: *Gua Sha* for Edema

One useful method for eliminating edema is called *gua sha* on your spleen meridian, especially the Sanyinjiao point and Yinlingquan point on your legs. These points are very effective for dealing with edema (fig. 61).

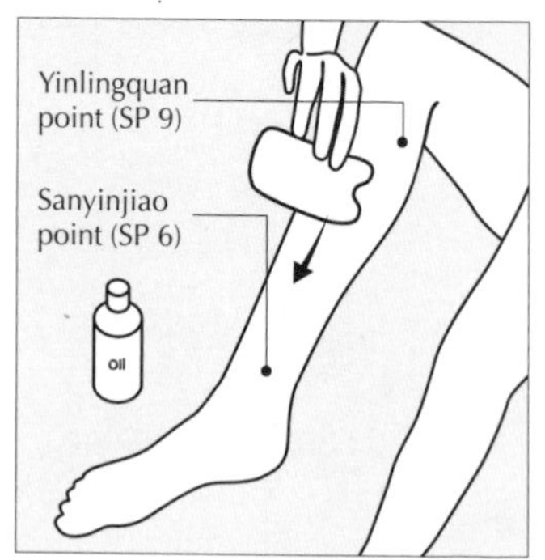

Fig. 61 The Location of Sanyinjiao point and Yinlingquan point

Steps:

1.Begin by massaging these points with your fingers for approximately two minutes. Massage in small circles clockwise and anti-clockwise for one minute each.

2.Afterwards use the *gua sha* board down your leg on the spleen meridian with a gentle to medium strength. Repeat approximately 100 times.

3.The next step is to hold your calf muscle and squeeze up and down the leg (your fingers will be strategically placed on your stomach meridian and your thumb will be on the spleen meridian lines as you massage up and down the leg.

Tips:

Gua sha is a wonderful technique, but it is not for everybody. Those who do not feel relaxed when having a treatment or don't feel any better afterwards don't need it.

It is important to be aware that *gua sha* can produce bruises, which may not be appreciated by everyone. Those with weak platelets or scar constitution may not be suited to this form of treatment as it may leave permanent marks for these individuals.

Also care should be taken when using *gua sha* on the sides of the neck where there are important arteries, too much *gua sha* on these areas could disturb your heart. If you are worried, then massage, acupressure, food remedies may be more appropriate.

If you choose to do *gua sha*, you should work with a professional since some caution is advised. While it is a very useful tool, *gua sha* is time consuming. For instance, when using *gua sha* on your back, you may need to do it 300 times to get any sort of benefit. This can make it slightly impractical unless you have someone who can administer it for you.

The face is less time consuming and only requires about 20–30 strokes in each area to be effective. Make sure you use a jade or stone *gua sha* board and gentle pressure. It can be very useful in reducing wrinkles and lifting sagging skin.

2) Imbalance: Cellulite

Cellulite occurs when invisible phlegm or dampness accumulates in a certain part of the body and gets stuck below the skin in the muscle area, according to TCM. You don't have to be overweight to have it, as it is not necessarily weight related, and it's accompanied by the declined function of kidney or spleen qi, and/or yang deficiency.

If the cellulite is occurring on the backs of your legs, it may be linked to your kidney system. Tonifying kidney qi and working on the related meridians with massage, *gua sha*, or acupressure may be effective.

External Remedies:

- Safflower oil is red in color and warming. It can reduce swollen legs. Safflower oil also strengthens the blood, promotes circulation, and treats dry skin.
- Orange oil diluted in a carrier oil. Orange oil enters the lung and stomach meridians to regulate energy flow, movement, and direction.

The following foods are recommended:

- Mustard seeds are hot and spicy and enter into the stomach and lung meridians. They are a perfect tonic to support the lung and spleen systems. They can be added to food or used to create a tea. Use 3–6 g of ground mustard seeds, boiled in 100 ml of water and consume as a tea. You may continue to add more hot water to your mustard seeds throughout the day. Some people have allergies to mustard seeds so make sure you monitor how you feel and always listen to your body.
- Eating fresh fig can help to speed up metabolism of water and fat. You can eat two to three fresh figs each day throughout

the year. The dried ones have a lot of sugar so fresh is best.

- Drinking Tieguanyin tea, a top quality Oolong tea that comes from Fujian province, is also very useful to help shift cellulite.
- Chia seed leaf, twig, and flower is also used in China for cellulite. It can be mixed with malt sugar to create a syrup.

3) Imbalance: Overweight

There are many reasons why people become overweight. Weight gain can be caused by specific illnesses, low thyroid, and hormone problems. For these specific issues, we recommend that you work together with your practitioner.

Other people gain weight due to emotional eating, or always feeling hungry due to being in a sub-healthy state. For instance, fatty liver is one condition that is at first caused by eating too much late and night, unhealthy food choices, or choosing foods that do not suit your particular constitution, It also contributes towards feeling sub-par.

The following foods are recommended:

- One method for dealing with excess weight is to control

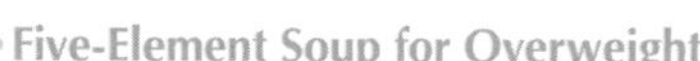

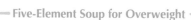

Five-Element Soup for Overweight

This soup is also very good for those who are obese with acne, lumps and constipation.

Ingredients: 75 g radish, 36 g burdock (optional 36 g aloe), 60 g carrots, 3 medium-sized shiitake mushrooms, 15 g radish leaf (optional 15 g corn), 2 L of water

How to Prepare?

1. Wash all the ingredients and cut them into bite size pieces.
2. Use an enamel pot to boil all the ingredients with water, then let simmer for one hour.
3. Eat the solid, then divide the soup into six portions.
4. Drink two bowls per day for three days, storing the left-over soup in glassware.
5. Take for two weeks.

inappropriate or excess hunger. You may use hawthorn berry for this purpose. Use 2 g of hawthorn berry powder with 2 g of green tea powder once a day for two weeks. This will help to cool the stomach and reduce hunger. If you already have symptoms of a cold stomach, then you can increase the proportion of hawthorn to 4 g and cook it together with 2 g of green tea. You can also choose fresh, uncooked hawthorn berries and eat two before each meal.

- Adding radish to your diet is another way to help you manage your weight.

4) Imbalance: Underweight

Being underweight can be caused by digestive weakness and poor absorption of your nutrients. This may be caused by either yin weakness or yang weakness.

Those who are underweight due to a yang weakness are more likely to have an aversion to cold, a pale complexion, and a stomach cannot take anything cold (for instance after eating something cold they may instantly get diarrhea or a stomach ache).

The following foods are recommended for yin weakness:

- Eat 30 g dried lychee each time in soup.
- Lentils can strengthen the spleen and stomach and help you to produce more digestive enzymes so you can more easily absorb your nutrition. They can also help to reduce diarrhea.

The following foods are recommended for yang weakness. These three are all good tonics for yang deficiency. A dosage of 1.5 to 3 g can be taken in a tea form or added to meals:

- Nutmeg warms the internal system and is good for a cold constitution. It warms and regulates the movements of the digestive system to prevent bloating pain, poor appetite, and vomiting. Nutmeg can reduce diarrhea in weak and cold constitutions. In TCM practice, nutmeg is particularly used to treat early morning diarrhea. Please note that too much nutmeg can be poisonous.

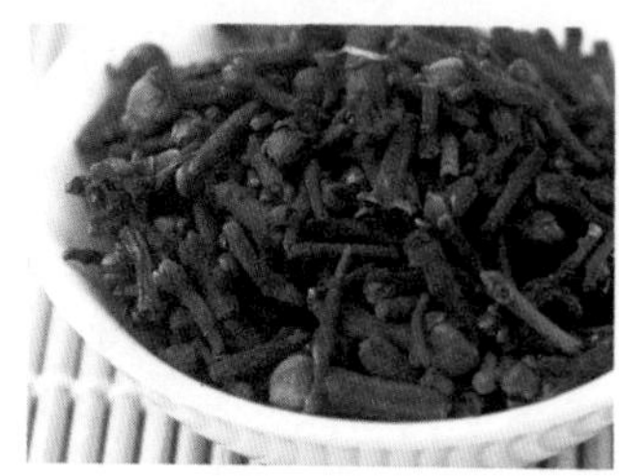
Fig. 62 Cloves

- Cloves (fig. 62) are effective for counteracting coldness in the body and the stomach. In addition to warming and calming the stomach and gastric area, they can be used to ease nausea, hiccups, and diarrhea, especially for infants and children.
- Fennel and fennel seeds dispel and counteract coldness by warming the internal body. They regulate qi and provide relief from pain, abdominal pain, and pain associated with hernias. They can regulate the motion of the stomach to prevent gas produced in the digestive system.

5) Imbalance: Saggy Skin

Saggy skin occurs when the energy of your body is sinking down inappropriately. Our bodies face a constant battle against gravity. This is most noticeable in our skin and muscles. When we are young, our energy is sufficient to combat gravity's pull. However, we might start to notice sagging skin as our energy begins to decline in older age.

It is very important to support the energy movements within your body in order to maintain a healthy appearance and to avoid sagging skin. The spleen energy should go up and stomach energy should go down. Furthermore, kidney energy should rise to meet the energy in the heart.

If your energy becomes weak or deficient, and/or the energy movements within the body begin to become disordered, then the organs cannot send up energy to our face and head. Stress and fatigue propagated by a fast lifestyle, too much junk food, aging, operations, and abortions can all disturb the energy patterns within your body.

Once the energy becomes weak, it begins to sink down and

this can be problematic for your skin and muscles. Furthermore, the spleen's function of "holding" is important in helping our muscles resist gravity.

The following foods are recommended:

- Astragalus root can be very effective to combat weak energy that sinks down. It can help to tonify qi and lift spleen yang. It targets the spleen and lung organ systems and is commonly used in China for prolapsed organs. Astragalus root can be purchased in granule form or as a ready-made herbal tincture and should be taken as prescribed by your

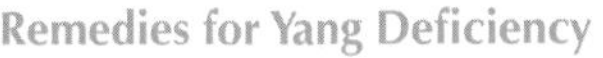

Remedies for Yang Deficiency

Yang energy is very important for creating a radiant complexion. Without sufficient yang energy, your face, hair, skin, and eyes will not glow.

If you consume a lot of cold foods and beverages, you may age more quickly. Your yang also energy helps to keep joints in good function and is important for longevity.

If you are yang deficient, you need to do the below things:

- Firstly, remove anything that may exasperate yang deficiency, such as a lot of cold foods and beverages, becoming too tired too often, overwork with no rest, and not eating or sleeping properly. These things make it difficult to regenerate your yang energy.
- Secondly, you should add specific foods and teas that tonify yang. If you have yang deficiency in a particular organ, you should add specific remedies that also enhance yang in the organ.
- Exercise in the sun can be especially good for tonifying yang. The sunlight is yang in nature and provides yang energy for your body. Vitamin D from the sun further benefits your system by helping your body produce energy.
- Sunlight boosts serotonin levels and happy chemicals in your body. Have you ever noticed that when you feel happy, you have a lot of energy and can complete many tasks without feeling tired? However, when you feel depressed, even one chore feels like a drag. Depression can be caused by stagnated energy, but can also cause energy in your body to become blocked, so sunlight can be a very useful tonic to counteract this.

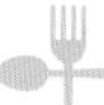

How to Take Astragalus Root

- Take 5 g astragalus root in granule form in hot water and drink as a tea.
- Make a decoction. Use 15 to 30 g, add 250 to 500 ml water, cook for 20 minutes. Remove the liquid, add 200 to 400 ml more fresh water, and boil for another 20 minutes. Add both batches of liquid together and drink throughout the day for three weeks.
- Add astragalus root to chicken soup. Ten small pieces or six large pieces could be cooked in the chicken broth. You could also combine it with 3–6 g of Bugbane Rhizome (Rhizoma Cimicifugae, *sheng ma*) to make it more effective.

own practitioner.

External remedies:

- Use dried ginger and cook it in water for 20 minutes. Once the liquid is warm enough, immerse a face cloth in the liquid and place it on the area of concern. After ten minutes, remove the face cloth from the skin. The heat on the skin can help to stimulate the collagen and may result in firmer skin.

Terrific Tummy

The meridian that travels down the center of your tummy area is the Ren meridian (Conception Vessel), moving from the centerline outwards, the kidney has two meridians running parallel to the Ren meridian, according to Chinese medicine. Moving out further still are the stomach meridians, and out again are the spleen meridians, and finally the liver meridians. In order to have a terrific tummy, there needs to be a smooth flow of energy and harmony between these meridians and their related organs (fig. 63).

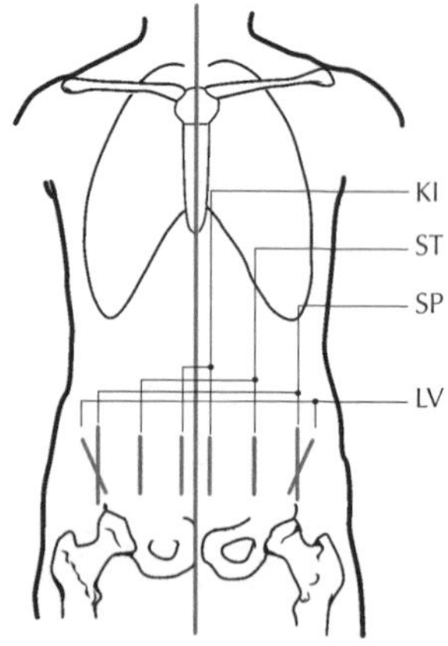

Fig. 63 The Ren meridian (Conception Vessel) and the parallel meridians

1) Imbalance: Constipation

While we know constipation makes it difficult to pass bowel movements, it can also cause you to accumulate toxins. This might cause your body to function less optimally. Constipation can occur in someone with a hot constitution or a cold constitution.

Those with a hot constitution may naturally be more yang. They may be outgoing and social, and love banquets. Their love for food may cause them to overindulge and they may be hindered by the fact that the food is not passing through easily.

Constipation in someone with a cold constitution is more likely caused by a yang deficiency. Those who have a yang deficiency may be already too yin. Those who have a yin constitution may be more introverted and avoid going out too often. Their constipation may not be caused by over indulging in banquets, but more likely a lack of yang energy. This person would be more likely to suffer from edema and cellulite. Some could be overweight.

The following foods are recommended:

- Cassia seed tea is good for those who are overweight and suffering from constipation. Take one teaspoon of whole or powdered cassia seeds for tea. Pull hot water with cassia seeds, water can be added each time. Please note that if you have more than two bowel movements within a day, you should reduce the dosage to 2/3 of a teaspoon. Don't overuse this method; continue for one week or until you feel better.
- Walnuts (for constipation due to yang deficiency) are warm and sweet and enter the kidney, lung, and large intestine meridians. They are effective for relieving constipation by moistening and nourishing the large intestine, and helping to treat dry stools especially when suffering from a slow moving colon. Similarly, they are suggested for people experiencing tightness when passing a stool, and perspiration or shortness of breath after bowel movements.
- Pine nuts are warm and sweet in nature and benefit the

liver, lung, and large intestine meridians. Pine nuts can treat dry conditions and promote the production of body fluid and blood. They also warm and regulate the bowels, treat a dry cough, and constipation that is caused by weakness. Furthermore, they nourish the blood, body fluids, and can help prevent and treat loose flesh and fatigue.

2) Imbalance: Bloating

There are many reasons why you may become bloated. Some bloating can occur as a result of food intolerances or indigested food fermenting in the intestines.

For instance, beans and root vegetables can have a high quantity of starch and anti-nutrients that prevent you from digesting them. You should always therefore soak beans, grains, and some seeds in order to aid in their digestion. You might also keep the proportion of the whole grains you consume down to only 20% of your grain intake as they are more difficult to digest.

Cruciferous vegetables may also be responsible for causing excess gas in the digestive tract.

TCM divides gas into two categories. Gas that goes up is caused by a disturbance in the stomach and gas that goes down is usually related to the spleen or colon.

The following foods are recommended:

- To treat the colon and regulate the spleen, you might use betelnut's peel 5 g to create a tea. Rose bud tea is another fabulous remedy.
- To treat the stomach, you could use remedies that reduce gas production like dried tangerine skin to into a tea (fig. 64).
- Food allergies, food poisoning, skipping meals, and eating big meals late at night can damage

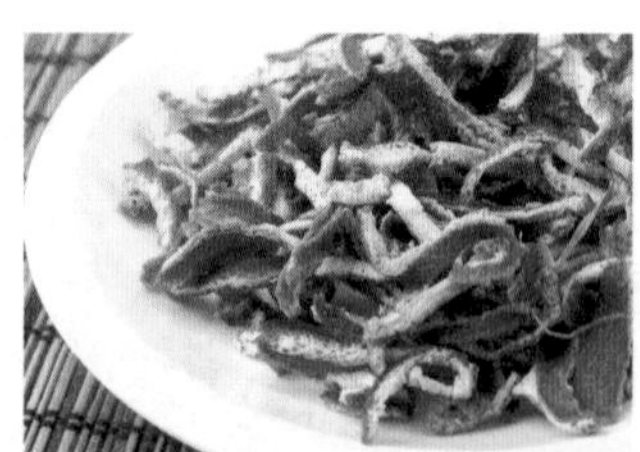

Fig. 64 Tangerine skin

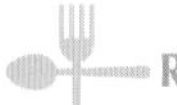

Recipe: Healing Rice Cakes

Ingredients for rice cakes: 100 g of glutinous rice, 150 g of normal rice, 500 ml of water, 15 g of licorice root (serves 5 people)
Ingredients for date paste: 30 to 60 dates, 50 to 100 ml water
How to Prepare?

1. Soak the two kinds of rice overnight or for at least half a day. Keep the soaking water for further use.
2. Separately add 30–60 dates to 50–100 ml water and boil it down to a paste.
3. Boil 350 ml of water with 15 g of licorice root.
4. Cook the rice using the licorice root water and rice soaking water.
5. Set the cooked rice in molds. Fill the inside of with the date paste and enclose with more rice.
6. Steam the cakes.

the delicate lining of the intestine. To heal the lining, you can make a tea or soup with jujubes and licorice's root, which are both very healing for the digestive tract. You may use six jujubes and 3 g of licorice root to make a decoction. Drink the liquid and eat the jujubes. Alternatively, you may add both these ingredients to chicken soup or a rice pudding.

3) Imbalance: Diarrhea

Diarrhea is often caused by a weak or over-stimulated digestive system, or food sensitivities. This could be caused by a spleen or kidney weakness.

Before using the remedies below, we recommend that you check that you do not have a more serious disease like colitis or dysentery if you are regularly experiencing diarrhea. If you are cleared of more serious diseases, then you can use the remedies listed below.

- Red bayberry (*yang mei*) wine can be a useful tonic to help chronic diarrhea.
- Pomegranate skin (juiced together with the fruit) or dried

pomegranate skin as a tea decoction (10 g) for two to three days can be very helpful. The skin is the most powerful part of this remedy.

- Dark plum (mume fruit) properties are neutral and it is sour and astringent. It enters the liver, spleen, lung, and large intestine channels. It is very good for relieving diarrhea as it works in the large intestine channel. Actually, this is one of the most commonly used herbs to treat chronic diarrhea that is caused by a deficiency of healthy qi.

Fresh Breath and Luscious Lips

Two common causes of bad breath can be caused by bacterial imbalances in your stomach such as H Pylori or by fermented food that has become stuck in your stomach.

We will now focus on two conditions that affect the beauty of your lips. The first is a change of color such as pale or purple lips, and the second is cracked and bleeding lips during certain dry seasons.

1) Imbalance: Bad Breath

There are many herbs in TCM that can help to unblock stomach qi and allow stagnated food to move down into the colon.

The following foods are recommended:

- Radish is neutral-cool, spicy, and sweet. It enters the spleen, stomach, lung, and large intestine meridians. Radish and its seeds are very good for removing food stagnation in helping to aid the function of the digestive system. They are excellent for relieving indigestion and dispelling distension. They can also help abnormally ascending qi to descend. In fact, radish and its seeds also help to regulate the movements of qi. It is used to treat a cough, wheezing, fullness and pressure in the chest, and lack of appetite. Add radish to meat soups, eat in salad, or consume them in Five-Element soup. The Five-Element soup was mentioned earlier and can detoxify the body, help achieve ideal weight goals, can prevent tumour growth.

- Pei lan orchard (Herba Eupatorii) is neutral in property, spicy in taste, and can remove dampness from the body by waking up the spleen. Sometimes the spleen gets lethargic due to accumulated dampness and the aromatic nature of pei lan orchard can help to stimulate the spleen. It can be made into a tea and is very effective for dealing with bad breath caused by fermentation of food in the stomach.
- You can also try chewing dried, raw green tea to refresh your breath or swishing some green tea in your mouth.

2) Imbalance: Pale or Purple Lips

Pale lips can be remedied by using food or herbal tonics for the blood. Purple lips, especially when combined with purple nails, can be caused by poor circulation to your extremities. It could also be caused by a blockage of mucus in your lungs.

The following foods are recommended for purple lips:

- Fresh gingko nuts are very effective for unblocking and improving lung function. Boil ten pieces of gingko nuts in water for three minutes then open the shell and eat the nut. You could also bake the nuts with salt. Once baked you can

Radish and Tofu Soup

Ingredients: 100 g of radish, 5–9 g of radish seeds (place the seeds inside a cotton bag), 100 g tofu, 2 g spring onion, 5 g of oil, 5 g salt, 300 ml of water and 1 tsp of sesame oil

How to Prepare?

1. Stir-fry the radish with oil for one to two minutes.
2. Add water and the seeds and bring to the boil. Stew the soup for 20 minutes.
3. Add tofu and boil again for five more minutes.
4. Add spring onion, salt and sesame oil (or you may substitute olive oil instead).

peel off the shell and eat. You could also add them to stir-fries or include them in sweet puddings.

- If you can't find the nuts, you could use gingko leaf powder or tablets (fig. 65). If you are just taking it for circulation to the lips, then you could take ½ the recommended dosage.

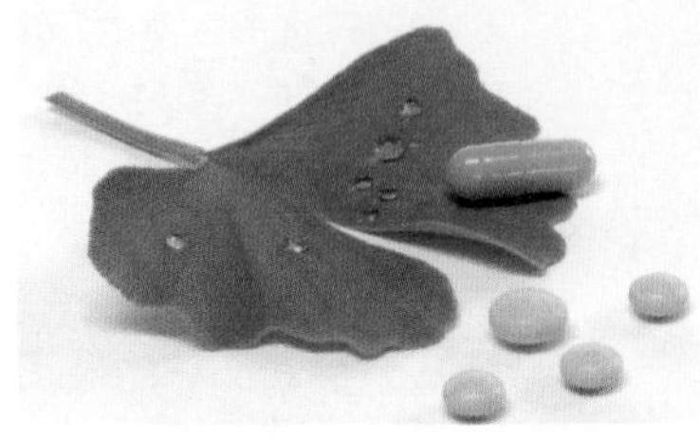
Fig. 65 Gingko leaf, powder and tablets

The following foods are recommended for pale lips:

- Wood ear may be rehydrated then stir-fried with any root vegetable like Chinese yam. It can also be added to chicken soup. A dosage of 5 g a day for ten days can be very helpful for combatting pale lips.

3) Imbalance: Cracked Lips or Canker Sores

Dehydration can lead to cracked lips. This can make the immune system in the lip area more vulnerable to canker sores or mouth ulcers. When dehydration progresses, an empty heat could develop, creating a condition more susceptible to mouth ulcers or canker sores.

The following remedies are recommended:

- Watermelon skin powder can be bought in any pharmacy in China. It is very effective for these conditions.
- You can use the light green part of the watermelon just under the skin. You could eat it raw or consume it as a pickle. If you would like to make a pickle, you should slice it and soak it in salt for 20 minutes. Squeeze the salty juice off and eat the pickle. You could also stir-fry it (including the white part) with a little bit of olive oil and add vinegar or sugar. You may also dry it in the sun or in a dehydrator, then soak 10 g before adding it to hot water to make a tea.

You could also add a teaspoon of honey.

- Eating a spoonful of olive oil and putting it on the lips is another remedy for cracked lips.
- Rehydrate a few wolfberries in a little hot water, mash it, and put it on your lips for 20 minutes before rinsing off.

4) Imbalance: Under Eye Bags

The following remedies are recommended:

- You could use an ice towel or some sliced cucumber to speed up circulation.
- Bags under the eyes can be treated by massaging the area. Using vitamin E oil, massage under the eye along the bone from the nose out to the temple with a medium pressure for 20 seconds.
- You can also perform the following facial muscle exercises. Open your mouth to make a small "O" shape as you tighten the area beneath the eyes by squinting your eyes (as if you are trying to read something that you can't see at a distance). Keep this expression for two to four seconds. Repeat a few times each night. Continue for a week or ten days to see some improvement.

So, your amazing spleen works tirelessly to help you break down your food and derive enough nourishment from what you eat. It sends valuable energy to all the digestive organs so that they can perform their duties effectively. It begins the process of producing qi, blood, and body fluids, which are all vital for your survival. It governs the blood within your vessels and performs the function of "ascending the clear". A healthy spleen system will contribute towards beautiful muscles, the prevention of water retention and cellulite, and will help you have a lovely figure. Looking after your spleen system will help you nourish a body that can last a lifetime.

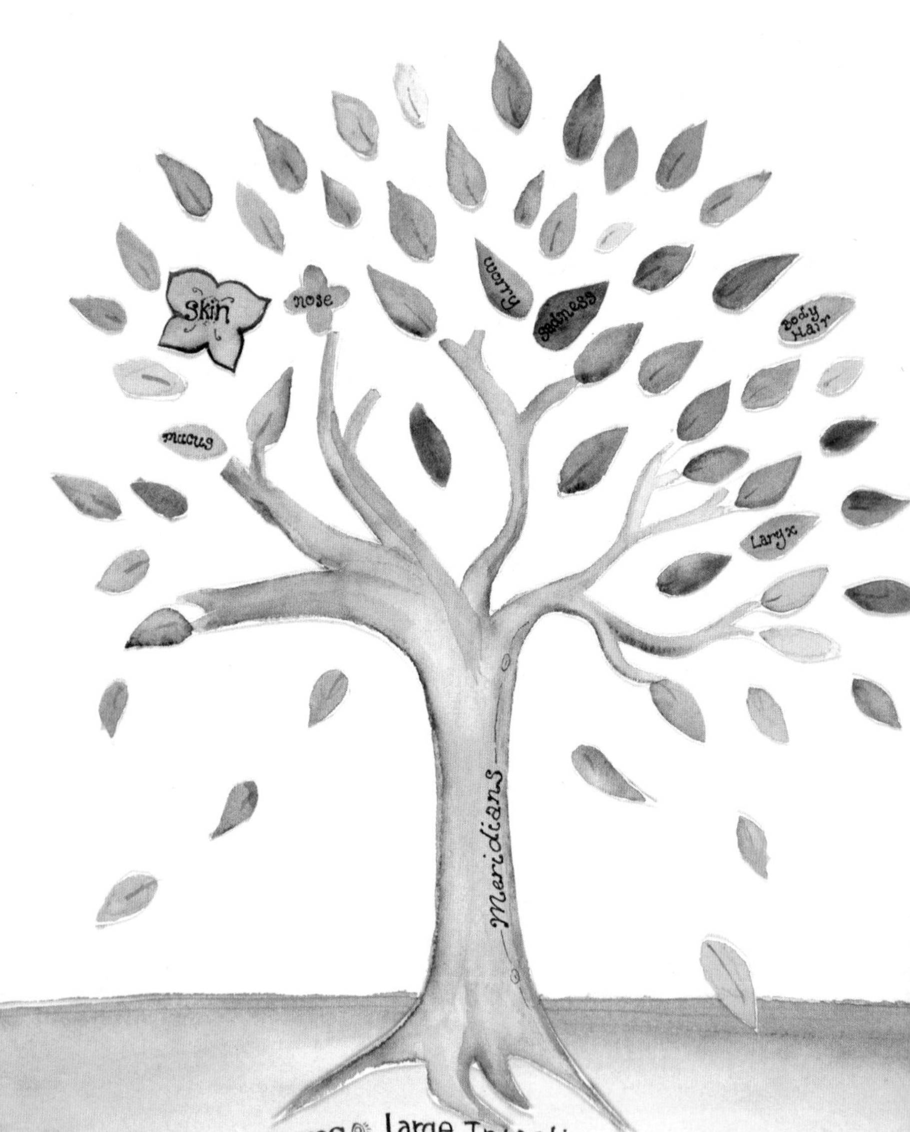
worry
sadness
Skin
nose
Body Hair
mucus
Laryx
Meridians
Lung & Large Intestine
worry & sadness

Chapter Eight

The Lung System

Roots

- *Zang*-organ: lung
- *Fu*-organ: large intestine
- Emotions of sadness and worry

Trunks and Branches

- Meridians: Taiyin Lung Meridian of Hand, Yangming Large Intestine Meridian of Hand

Leaves

- Lustrous body hair
- Protective mucus in the nose (suitable amount)
- Larynx with sonorous voice

Fruits

- Emotions of sadness and worry (also part of the "roots" system)

Flowers

- Gorgeous hydrated and blemish free skin
- Well ventilating nose with a keen sense of smell

Left Fig. 66 The lung system tree

1. Basic Facts about the Lung System

The lung and large intestine organs are the roots of lung system. Nutrition and qi is delivered to the extremities by the lung and large intestine meridians. The skin, body hair, larynx, mucus in the nose and nose are all related to the lung system and you can tell how healthy your lung system is by observing disharmony in these areas.

The lung is the organ that is responsible for governing and regulating the body's qi through breath, it also helps controlling the circulation of blood, and regulating the body's metabolism of fluid, according to the *Yellow Emperor's Canon*.

The emotions of sadness and worry are also connected to the lung.

2. Functions of the Lung

In ancient times, Chinese people used analogies from nature and social structure to help people understand the inner workings of the human body. The *Yellow Emperor's Canon* is a very famous book and it describes the heart as the emperor, the liver as the general, and the lung as the prime minister of the body.

In TCM, the lung has many different functions.

Body's First Line of Defense

The lung is the first line of defense in your body. It works hard to protect the other organs. In terms of location within the human physique, the lung is located higher than any of the other organ systems. In order to explain why the lung was higher up in the chest cavity than the heart (since the heart is the emperor) during ancient times, the *Yellow Emperor's Canon* described the lung as the "umbrella" or "canopy" for the heart. By using this analogy, it is easy to make reference to the protective features of the lung. If anything invades the body, like a bacteria or virus, the lung will fight them first. However, they may also be the first to suffer.

The lung is quite delicate as there are many small chambers called alveoli within the lung structure that do not like to be too hot, cold, or blocked. It has self-protective and self-cleaning mechanisms. The nose acts as a filter and there are many small hairs (cilia) and mucus that lines the inside of the breathing tubes in order to help remove debris and keep foreign bodies out.

Governing Respiration

The function of governing respiration is particularly related to the inhalation of air. Your lung is the intermediary organ between your internal body and the external environment. When you inhale, your lung qi should go down (descending) and in. When you breathe out, your lung qi should go up and out (dispersing). In this way, the process of respiration influences all the qi movements within the body.

Proper breathing is essential for the lung system and also the entire body. As we know, oxygen is used in different physiological functions and is essential to survival. Any kind of disturbance to breathing will eventually affect the whole body.

Almost immediately after birth, a baby will take his or her first breath. Respiration is a natural process that requires no planning or thinking. As we get older, however, we often begin to develop disordered breathing patterns, such as shallow breathing and holding the breath when we are stressed or completing a difficult task.

These incorrect breathing patterns can affect the lung qi. It also affects the total amount of qi within your system. This is one reason why meditation can be an important tool for regulating your breathing and affecting your health.

Breathing properly also helps to regulate your sympathetic

and parasympathetic nervous system, further promoting whole body health. Deep and diaphragmatic breathing helps you move from a sympathetic nervous system state (fight and flight) to a parasympathetic nervous system state (rest and digest). Shallow breathing and patterns of holding stress further encourages a hyper-sympathetic nervous system condition and contributes towards the over-production and over-use of hormones such as cortisol and adrenaline.

Regulating Body Fluid

The lung regulates the waterways and facilitate water metabolism. This function is linked to the ascending and descending feature of the lung.

When lung qi goes up and out, the body fluids will follow and find their way to your face, mouth, and head. When the body fluids go out to the skin's surface, they can provide essential nourishment to moisten your muscles and skin. Therefore, the lung governs the upper-stream (the areas from the chest to the head including the upper limbs) of water metabolism.

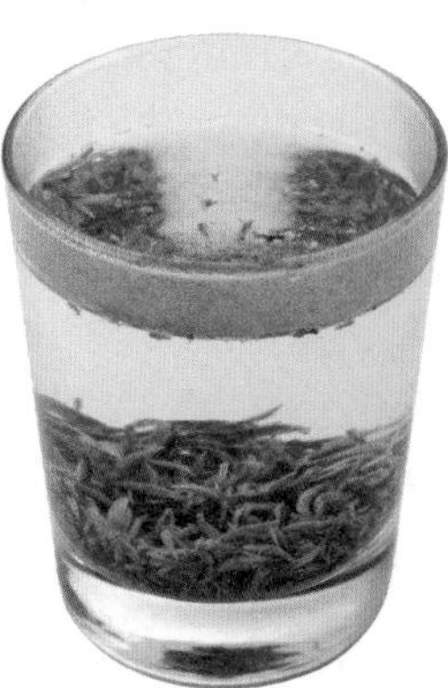

Fig, 67 Green tea is good for regulating body fluid.

A disturbance in lung qi caused by body fluids that cannot follow the ascending function of coming up and out may result in dryness or water accumulation in the upper-stream. Dryness might be observed in the skin, mouth, and nose. When body fluids become stuck in the throat or chest, they can transform into phlegm, excess mucus, or water retention. This can also impact the large intestine, since it is joined to the lung via meridians. It may also impact the urinary system (fig. 67).

The function of the lung in water metabolism is important since it also helps to govern whether you can sweat properly or not. If you do not sweat properly, you may not be ridding the body of toxins and excess wastewater. If you sweat too much, you might experience weakness and dry skin due to a lack of body fluids.

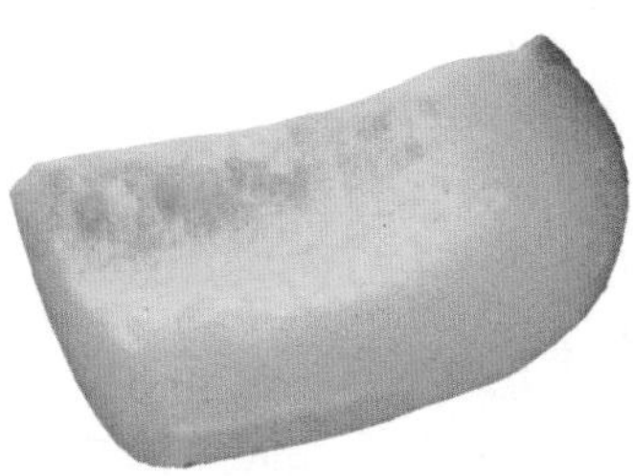

Fig. 68 Winter melon is slightly cold in temperature, sweet, and bland in taste. It can produce body fluids and remove toxins.

So lung qi should be able to adequately direct the body fluids to the surface of the skin to nourish the skin, nerves, and muscles, and then expel wastewater through sweating, the urinary system, and the colon in appropriate amounts (fig. 68).

Water Retention and the Related Organs

Many organs can influence water retention.

Water retention in the upper body might be related to the lung, in the middle it may be related to the spleen, and in the lower abdomen excess fluids might be related to the kidney.

If you are experiencing swelling in legs, you might investigate and see if you have other symptoms relating to the spleen or kidney. Swelling in the face, eyes, fingers, arms, or even scalp might be related to the lung due to inadequate fluid metabolism.

Facilitating Convergence of the Blood Vessels

All the blood vessels have junction in the lung. Traditionally, the lung were referred to as the meeting point of "one hundred vessels".

The breathing process of the lung can bring fresh qi to transform waste blood into fresh blood. Then heart and lung qi will distribute the fresh blood to the whole body. Breathing helps to expel waste products, including the breathing that occurs through skin, mouth, and nose.

Governing Qi

Lung qi is vital to support all of the functions of the lung. It guides the process of inhaling oxygen and exhaling carbon dioxide. Having enough oxygen in your blood is very important for health and energy production. So the process of transforming qi can play a vital role in how energetic you feel. If you lung is working optimally, they will facilitate the transformation of oxygen and nutrition into qi.

The lung is very important to defensive qi. If your lung works optimally, defensive qi will be sent to the surface of your body, including your skin and the area just below your skin.

In addition, the qi in each organ system will flow in the correct direction. For instance, stomach qi will descend, spleen qi will ascend, and heart and kidney qi will cooperate and harmonize with each other. The heart is especially reliant on qi for its own mental and physical functions. Every part of your body including your brain craves oxygen and cannot function without it.

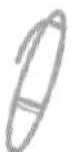

The Chinese Concept of Qi

In traditional Chinese culture, qi is a fundamental concept and it is a part of everything that exists. It is everywhere in all the wonders of the universe. Everything you can see, feel, and experience contains qi.

Where does Qi Come from?

Qi is created from oxygen that is inhaled during the breathing process, food essence, and original qi that you are born with.

- The lung plays a very important role in this process because your breathing processes enrich your qi. Without good breathing habits, the quality and quantity of qi can be affected.
- Food essence comes from the TCM concept of the spleen which refers to the organs with digestive functions including the spleen, pancreas, and part of small intestine. The spleen transforms and transports your nutrients into "clear qi".
- You are born with an original qi and it is stored in your kidney.

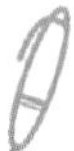

Names and Types of Qi

Why Qi has Different Names?

Once qi has been created, it is distributed to all the organs and meridians. Qi that ends up in the spleen is renamed as spleen qi, qi that ends up in the liver becomes liver qi and so forth.

Four Types of Qi

Qi can be further classified into four types:

- Nutrition qi (*ying qi*): It originates from nutrition of food transformed by the spleen and stomach. It is the component part within the blood flowing throughout the body. Nutrition qi circulates in the blood vessels, and is transformed into blood to nourish the whole body.
- Defensive qi (*wei qi*): It is produced mainly from the nutrients we absorb from food. The functions of defensive qi is protect your body against viruses, bacteria, cold, or anything that may cause harm to the body. Defensive qi is diffused under the skin. During the daytime, defensive qi surrounds the blood veins and meridians. At night, it goes into the organs. The lung regulates its movement under the skin.
- Original qi (*yuan qi*): It originates from congenital essence, also known as kidney qi. It is replenished and "topped up" by your nutrition after birth. However, it declines as you begin to age.
- Chest qi (*zong qi*): It originates mainly from the oxygen inhaled during exercise and from food essence. It is predominately stored in the Danzhong point between the lung and heart (fig. 69). Chest Qi keeps the airways open for the lung. If it can effectively flow to the throat, singing and talking for long periods of time without discomfort will be easy. For the heart, chest qi helps to warm the heart and promotes efficient blood circulation.

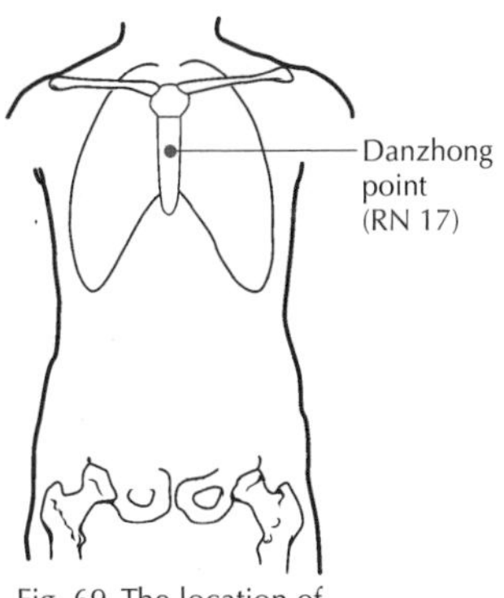

Fig. 69 The location of Danzhong point

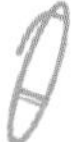

Relationship of Qi, Blood, and Body Fluids in the Lung

Qi, blood, and body fluids have a very special relationship in the lung area and are influenced by each other (fig. 70).

The following Chinese saying helps us understand this symbiotic relationship:

Qi produces blood and body fluid
Qi promotes blood and body fluid circulation
Qi controls blood and body fluid
Blood and body fluid carries qi
Blood and body fluid share the same source and help each other in times of need.

This healthy relationship begins in the lung and continues throughout the whole body. If this relationship is not formed properly in the lung or is blocked due to an accumulation of waste or another factor, then it can disturb this essential balance throughout your whole system.

The lung is a special place for the metabolism of qi, blood, and body fluids. Any issues with metabolism of these essential bodily substances may be caused by, and on a more positive note, helped by supporting the lung and changing the way you breathe. At times, qi deficiency might be caused by a lack of oxygen so improving lung function is essential.

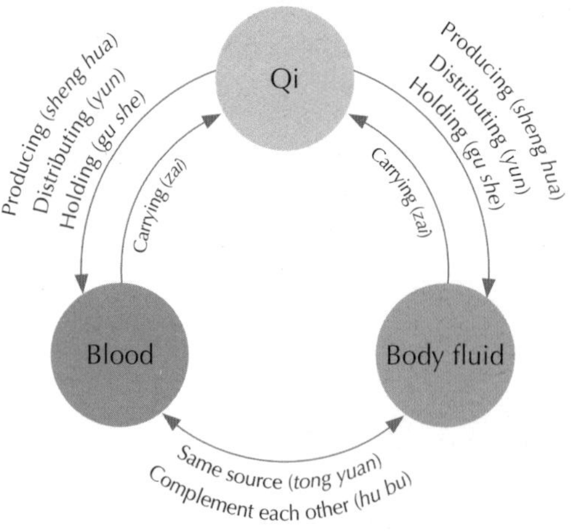

Fig. 70 Relationship between qi, blood and body fluid

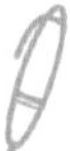

Factors that Affect the Lung Functions

Environmental conditions, negative emotions, and genetic factors can disrupt effective breathing. If this occurs, the descending and dispersing functions of lung qi can become disturbed.

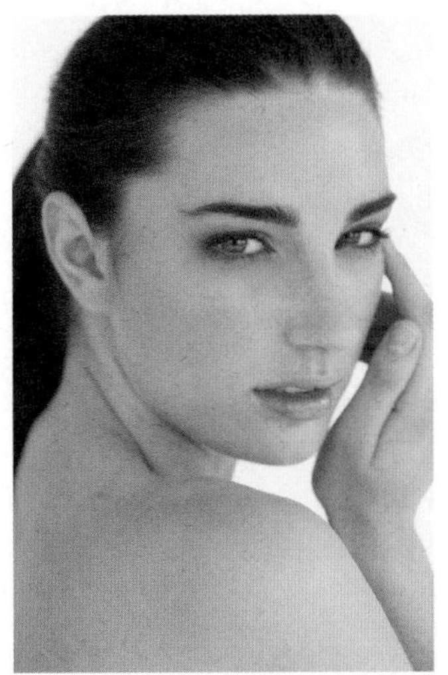

Fig. 71 Supporting and improving the lung system is good for your beauty.

- Environmental factors: These include bacterium, virus (germs), pollution, food intolerances, and allergies. They can create a buildup of mucus impairing lung function.
- Genetic factors: Some people are born with a stronger respiration system than others and there are certain and medical conditions that can inhibit natural breathing function. Asthma is an example of a condition that inhibits the airways and results in difficulty getting oxygen into the lung.
- Negative emotions: Controlling your mind and stress levels is important for a healthy lung system.

Doing exercises and breathing fresh air can improve lung function. Parents with children who suffer with lung issues should ensure that they take them into nature often. Regular exercise and movement is also important in developing lung qi that will be strong enough for adulthood (fig. 71).

3. Meridians of the Lung System

The deep points of the Taiyin Lung Meridian of Hand begin inside the stomach area and run down to connect with the large intestine. The lung meridian then passes through the diaphragm, then all the way to the lung. From here, it comes up the esophagus, travels up the back of the larynx to the throat. From the throat, it travels out towards both sides of the chest, then down along the ridges of the arms to the heel of the palm, and finally ends on the thumb.

The Taiyin Lung Meridian of Hand (fig. 72) and the Yangming Large Intestine Meridian of Hand (fig. 73) are linked together. The lung meridian is linked to the large intestine meridian, which begins from the tip of the index finger (on the side closest to the thumb), then follows the index finger up across the inside of the knuckle, up the back of the hand to the bone inside the wrist, up the forearm to the elbow, it then travels up the outside of the arm to the shoulder, and it enters the lung from here. It then travels up the side of the throat, then across to the base of the nose on the opposite side.

You can help both lung and colon function by rubbing or massaging along these meridian lines. If you find a painful area, spend a little more time massaging it.

The lung and large intestine are intimately connected. If the lung energy is able to adequately descend, then it will help the colon have good bowel motions. If the colon is functioning optimally, then lung qi will also move smoothly.

In clinical situations, it is often observed that if heat and mucus have accumulated in the lung then constipation of the colon may occur. If the colon has excess heat, it may damage and stagnate the qi's movement and can disturb the descending and dispersing functions of the lung. Ultimately, this may cause asthmatic breathing, cough, or chest fullness.

Due to this *zang-fu* relationship, you can affect one by treating the other in Chinese medicine. If you are experiencing trouble with your lung, you might gain relief by treating the large intestine and vice versa.

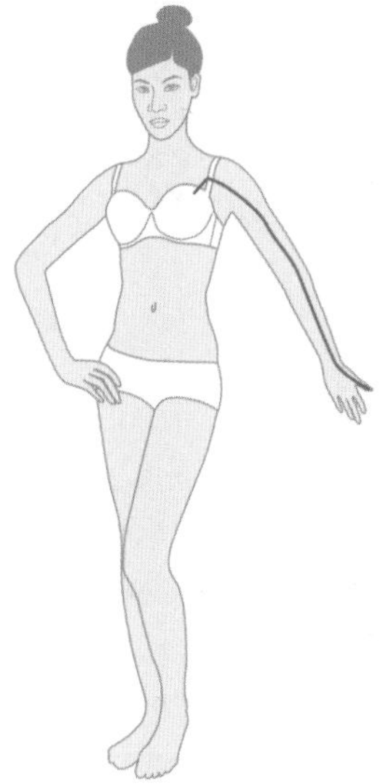

Fig. 72 Taiyin Lung Meridian of Hand

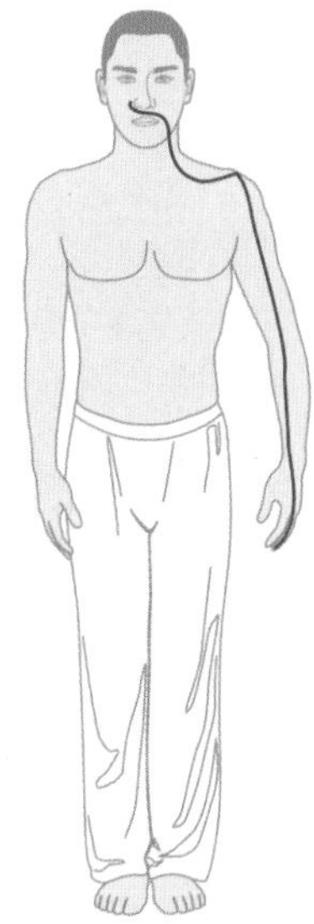

Fig. 73 Yangming Large Intestine Meridian of Hand

For instance, if you were constipated due to stagnation in the colon, doing some breathing exercises might help to relax it. If your lung were blocked with mucus or phlegm, having a bowel movement might help to clear some of this.

In the West, many people swallow phlegm rather than spit it out because we instinctively know that the phlegm will make its way out of the body via the colon. So, we also subconsciously realize that there is a link between the lung and the colon.

4. Lung System and Beauty

Beautiful skin, a healthy nose, and excellent fluid metabolism are reliant upon effective lung function.

Skin and Body Hair: Reflection of Lung Function

Both the skin and body hair depend on the lung's function of ascending. Defensive qi and body fluids make their way to the surface of your skin to nourish, hydrate, and provide warmth. Glowing and hydrated skin is a sign that your lung is functioning optimally.

Dry skin and the inability to sweat could indicate that body fluids are not making their way to your skin adequately, and defensive qi is not performing its function of opening and closing the pores properly to allow waste water to come out through the process of sweating. This could be caused by blockage of lung qi or a qi deficiency. Treatments might include unblocking or strengthening lung qi.

Someone who has too much spontaneous and continuous sweating may see an improvement in their symptoms by strengthening lung qi through food and herbal remedies.

Other conditions of the skin such as dry patches, summer rashes, peeling of the skin, and acne when you eat too many spicy foods all indicate that your skin is not adapting to different temperatures or you are eating foods that are disrupting your lung qi production and distribution. For any skin condition, think of the lung first.

The texture of your skin is not only dependent upon your heritage, but is deeply rooted in a healthy lung system. In TCM, the skin along with the muscles actually provide a very strong barrier for the immune system to protect the body against outside forces. Any time you suffer from a skin condition, it may indicate your defensive qi is weak and you should look after the lung. Normal lung function will ensure that the skin texture is smooth and evenly nourished, and free of conditions such as dry patches. The spleen and lung systems will cooperate together to ensure that your skin does not easily sag by providing elasticity and hydration.

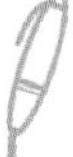

Defensive Qi and Skin

Defensive qi is very important to your skin health:

- It reinforces your skin's texture, and it warms, moistens, nourishes, and strengthens the skin and muscles.
- It helps the skin maintain a steady temperature.
- It also ensures the pores of the skin open and close appropriately. If someone is experiencing spontaneous or continuous sweating (without feeling hot), or has pores that are too open all the time causing an aversion to wind and cold, then this might be indicative that defensive qi is weak. Having chills or feeling very hot when it's not expected are further indications.
- Defensive qi also plays a role in keeping the muscles warm and strong. The lung regulates its movement under the skin and help to open and close the pores. Those who are prone to frequent colds may have both lung and defensive qi weakness.

Healthy skin will have rosy pink hues beneath the natural skin tone, which is an indication of good energy and blood flow. Soft, smooth, hydrated skin that remains firm indicates a balance of yin and yang.

Stretch marks after pregnancy are a sign that your skin does not have as much elasticity as it ought to and may require a little extra love.

Of course, no one has perfect skin, but we can all make the most of what we have and balance our inner terrain for a vibrant complexion. Having oily skin when you are young might cause your skin to be less prone to wrinkles later on. However, oily skin does increase the size of the pores. Dry skin might be more beautiful during youth, as the skin pores are small, but measures need to be taken to prevent it from wrinkling later on due to too much dryness. You can get a diagnosis for the type of skin you have, whether it be oily, dry, combination, hyper-allergenic, or neutral from a beauty therapist. Then you can harmonize your skin condition accordingly using internal and

Gardenia: the Chinese Foundation

In ancient China, gardenia was used as a foundation. The flower and the fruit were pressed through material similar to cheese cloth, and the yellow liquid was collected and dried in the sun. The powder was used as a foundation.

Dried gardenia flower powder can also be used externally to stop nosebleeds.

external methods.

Another factor about skin care in Asia is that Chinese people also don't tend to bake themselves in the sun for an entire day due to the fact that white skin is highly valued. But getting at least 20 minutes of sunshine in the summer and over an hour in the winter is a regular habit.

Your body hair also depends on defensive qi and body fluids for nourishment and growth. Excessive body hair is not really popular at this point in time. However, having some body hair is important for the functions of sweating and defense. Clinically, there are not many practical treatments to encourage the growth of body hair, but some hair is necessary and the lung governs its growth.

Nose: "Opening" of the Lung

The lung opens to the nose, just as the liver opens to the eyes. Your nose is an important tool for respiration and is also responsible for your ability to smell.

Oxygen comes into our body through the nose or mouth and as mentioned, it's vital for many body processes. Having a clear sinus passage is important because the nose has hairs to filter the air as it enters. Sinus conditions can cause you to breathe through the mouth more frequently, which does not have the same filtering function as the nose and may increase episodes of sore throats and bronchitis.

Many of us do not realize that your sense of smell is dependent upon lung function and the ability to smell is not just a process that occurs in the nose area.

In TCM, a blocked nose (any time of the day or night) and poor sense of smell may be treated by addressing lung function. These symptoms might indicate lung qi deficiency or disharmony in the descending and dispersing feature of the lung.

It is important that the lung's function of "ascending" sends qi and body fluids to the nose. Adequate moisture in the nasal cavity is important, but there should not be so much moisture that your nose becomes runny. If the nose is too dry inside or constantly runny, then you should treat your lung system.

Larynx: Passageway for Oxygen to Enter the Lung

In TCM, the larynx includes both the larynx and the tonsils, which both belong to the lung system. So when we discuss the larynx, we are including the tonsils. The larynx is responsible for helping send oxygen down to the lung after the nose has inhaled it. It is also viewed as a door for oxygen and your lung meridian is linked here.

At the same time, the larynx is an important organ for your voice. Smooth movements of qi to the larynx and a good strong voice are directly influenced by lung function.

The larynx is a protective barrier against outside pathogenic factors. As we already know, the tonsils play a role in protecting the body from illness, and this is often the first area to suffer, as your tonsils work hard to protect your lung.

In Chinese medicine, it is not recommended to remove the tonsils as is commonly practiced in Western medicine. Constant tonsillitis is not a sign that you should remove them. Rather, it is a sign that your tonsils are doing a very good job of protecting your lung from a greater sickness and evidence that you may need to strengthen your lung organ system.

Since your tonsils are the first line of defense against the outside world, you should do everything you can to strengthen them and take further measures to protect yourself from the elements such as cold weather. Supporting the lung would also treat a weak voice, hoarse voice, and sore throat.

The color of the mucus can indicate the condition of the lung. For instance, white, transparent or watery mucus might indicate lung coldness. Bleeding, yellowish, or greenish discharge indicates a hot condition in the lung.

Worry and Sadness: Emotions of the Lung

The fruit of the lung is the emotions of worry and sadness. More often than not, we worry about things that haven't happened and may never happen. It is a waste of energy and can rob us from the present moment. Sadness, on the other hand, usually occurs as a result of an event that has happened that you could not control. For instance, a loss of a loved one or inability to find a job.

Too much sadness and worry is not healthy and can cause a lot of disturbance to lung function. It also consumes a lot of lung qi. Crying and sadness will affect your breathing and can potentially affect the energy movements throughout your entire body.

TCM would treat the lung to help people deal with excess worry, particularly since many of the things we worry about will never come to pass. If the lung is already weak due to a physical illness, the body may have less tolerance for worrying and sad situations. This can then initiate a vicious cycle of more sadness and worry. Of course, there is a time and place for sadness. We are referring to chronic sadness and worry when we discuss its negative impact on lung function.

There are many stories of people experiencing serious lung

conditions after a very sad or troublesome event. For instance, you may have heard of someone developing lung cancer or pneumonia after an intensely traumatic or sad occurrence that they could not control. Deep sadness, especially if it is prolonged, can weaken the lung.

If you experience a very sad situation and are finding it difficult to move beyond these emotions, or find yourself constantly worrying, you could take proactive measures to strengthen and protect your lung during this stressful period. Gentle exercise, herbs, food remedies, massage, acupuncture, and developing good breathing habits can help support your lung. These strategies will also help improve your moods and influence your emotions.

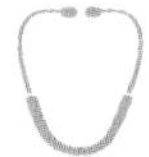

Autumn: Season to Strengthen the Lung System

Some people love autumn, when the leaves begin to change color, the sky becomes a little clearer, and there is less humidity. Many individuals find a greater sense of harmony in their physical body and a sense of well-being. Those who struggle in summer, due to feeling too hot or who regularly experience wind allergies, may find autumn to be a great relief. They may find themselves able to explore the outdoors more.

Some people actually begin to struggle in autumn. The dryness in the environment may instigate a dry cough, skin conditions, and a chronic runny nose. This group of people may find that their worries start to build up and they may struggle with unreasonable sadness. When they see the leaves falling, they may begin to feel a sense of loss, have feelings of loneliness, and may even begin to dread the upcoming winter. This group of people may do well to strengthen their lung system, especially before the season arrives.

In China, hospitals have many treatment protocols that are performed in summer to prevent bronchitis, asthma, runny nose symptoms, and other lung conditions that may occur in autumn for susceptible individuals. If you have any recurring conditions related to the lung that occur in autumn, it is wise to take a proactive approach and strengthen your body during the season before.

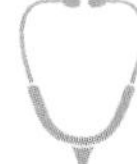

Case Study

Lin had a dry cough every autumn for three years in a row. She was encouraged by a TCM doctor to eat more almonds, silver ear, and lily bulbs several months before autumn arrived. She had 20 g every day during summer. The following autumn she was symptom free.

5. Beauty Problems and Enhancement

Through their dispersing function, the lung are responsible for sending body fluids and defensive qi to all the surfaces of the skin to warm, moisten, and nourish the skin cells. A weakness or disturbance in this function can cause many skin imbalances, nose, sinus and throat conditions.

Sensational Skin

In this section, we will discuss dry, sensitive, and pigmented skin. We will also discuss skin blemishes (such as warts, sores, raised lumps, and acne).

Chinese culture has some very special remedies that help to regenerate youthful skin and some TCM hospitals provide services using traditional anti-aging techniques and materials. Many clients have seen the reduction of wrinkles and pigmentation, and have even noticed some facial lifting after following a three-month protocol. They were treated with special Chinese facial massages accompanied with TCM herbal masks and nourishing creams (made almost exclusively from herbs and plants), prescribed herbal tonics, and followed certain food advice suited to their constitutions and imbalances.

1) Imbalance: Dry Skin

The following foods are recommended:

- Lily bulb can be cooked in a soup and is very good for dry skin. Noticeable results can be seen after three weeks of consuming this soup. It goes very nicely with silver ear or with pears, which are also fabulous tonics for the skin. You could also add a nut oil like pine nut oil in the soup.

External therapy:

- Cracked heels were often treated with lard in ancient times. In modern times, hemp seed oil is another good option.

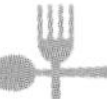

Silver Ear and Lily Bulb Soup for Dry Skin

This particular recipe is nourishing to the lung, helps to increase body fluid, quenches thirst, and moistens dry skin.

Ingredients: 30 g of silver ear, 500 ml of water, 60 g of lily bulb (fresh or dry), 3 tsp of honey

How to Prepare?

1.Presoak the dry silver ear or dry lily bulb.

2.Boil 500 ml of water then add the silver ear. Bring to the boil again and stew for ten minutes.

3.Add the lily bulb and stew for another half an hour.

4.Add honey before serving.

Treat kidney for Dry skin

Cherries are warm, sweet and sour. They can enter the spleen and kidney channels. Cherries are great to strengthen qi and nourish blood, which will provide a moisturizing effect on the skin. They can also help with vertigo and palpitations. A desert of cherries combined with silver ear can help to promote beautiful skin.

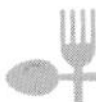

Treat Heart for Dry Skin

You could create a nourishing paste to counteract dry, dull looking skin, and wrinkles. Create a jam-like paste using 200 g of wolfberries, 250 g longan fruit, and water. Boil down into a paste and eat one teaspoon twice a day (morning and evening) on an empty stomach for one month.

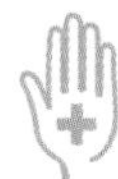

Chinese Facial Treatment

The Procedure

1.Clean your face with your cleanser.

2.Use a positive ion facial steamer for 5–10 minutes. If you don't have a facial steamer, put hot water in a bowl (you may use a few drops of your favorite essential oil if you like), place a towel over your head, and allow the steam to open your pores. Please use caution, as steam can be hot.

3.Dry your face. Then spritz it with some facial floral water or use a toner.

4.Place some cream or facial oil on your forehead, both cheeks, nose and chin.

5.Begin your pressure point and facial massage (see below steps).

6.Apply a mask (see below steps).

7.Spritz with floral water or tone.

8.Apply moisturizer.

Pressure Point and Facial Massage (Fig. 74)

1.Begin by massaging your forehead in upward brush strokes (massage up and out towards the hair-line).

2.Massage around the eyes in a circle. Begin from the inner eyebrow following the brow to the end of the eyebrow, down along the bone under the eye, then in towards the now and back up to the eyebrow.

3.Massage a half moon across the eyebrows (going in to out).

4.Massage a half moon from the nose out across the upper cheekbone.

5.Begin to stimulate the pressure points. Using your finger make small circular motions on each point for two minutes.

- Baihui point (DU 20): top of the head.
- Taiyang point (EX-HN 5): both temples.
- Yintang point (EX-HN 3): in between the eyebrows.
- Cuanzhu point (BL 2): just below the inner eyebrows.
- Yuyao point (EX-HN 4): middle of the eyebrow.
- Sizhukong point (SJ 23): end of the eyebrow.
- Jingming point (BL 1): inner corners of the eyes.
- Sibai point (ST 2): depression on upper cheek bone, in line with pupil.
- Yingxiang point (LI 20): approximately 0.5 mm away from nostril on both sides.

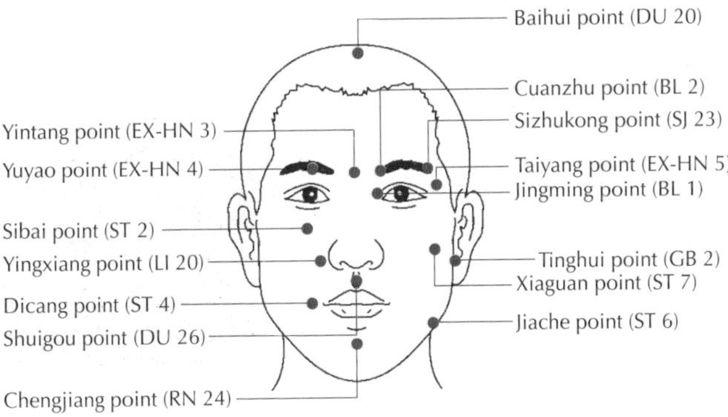

Fig. 74 Acupoints for facial massage

- Shuigou point (DU 26): in the crest between the nose and lips, about 1/3 of the way down from the nose.
- Dicang point (ST 4): 0.5 mm away from the corners of the mouth.
- Chengjiang point (RN 24): in the depression below the lower lip, the point is located on a small mound, if you can feel your teeth through your skin you are a little bit too high.
- Jiache point (ST 6): on the jaw line, you can feel the muscle move if you clench your teeth (both sides).
- Tinghui point (GB 2): the little crease where the face meets the ear, approximately half way down, if you open your mouth you will feel the little depression, close your mouth again, and massage the point.

The Masks

We have included two options here or you may use your own.

Option 1: For pigmentation, you could find a mask based on marine collagen.

Option 2: For detoxing your skin, increasing circulation, cooling heat, and to help clear pimples, you could use medical grade gypsum. Use 300 g of gypsum powder and mix it with water until you get a nice thick paste. Protect your eyebrows, mouth, and eyes with wet cotton pads, and your hair with a towel (This is an important step because the mask will harden and you don't want it to take your eyebrows with it when you remove it). Apply the paste to your whole face. Relax for 25–30 minutes, it will become solid once the mask cools. Remove the mask and clean the face.

2) Imbalance: Sensitive Skin

The following foods are recommended:

- Mung beans are cold in nature and sweet in taste. They enter through the heart, liver, and stomach channels. Mung beans can help to clear heat and toxins. They are especially good at removing toxic heat since they are cold in nature, and can help to treat carbuncles, sores, and may help sooth flare-ups and pain.

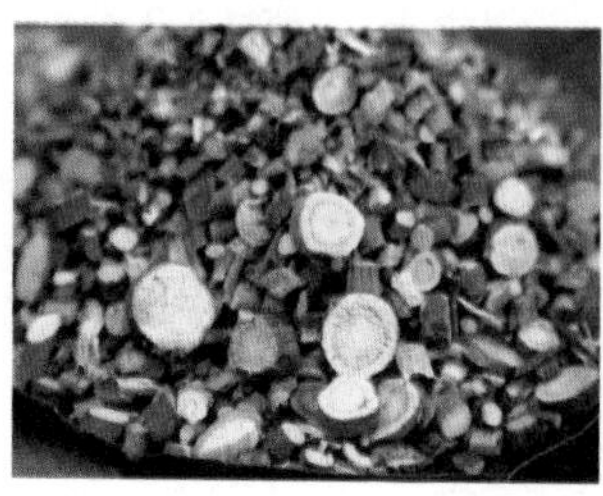

Fig. 75 Licorice roots

- You could make a tea with 3 g of licorice root (fig. 75).
- Fo-ti root is cooling and can calm heat conditions on the skin. It can be cooked and applied on the sensitive area to nourish the skin and bring blood flow.
- Honey is neutral, slightly sweet, and enters the lung, spleen, and large intestine channels. Honey is very nourishing and moistening to the lung system. It can help to ease constipation and dry skin.

External remedies:

- You could apply honey directly on the skin to treat scalds, burns, and to help clear toxins, reduce swelling, and itchiness caused by bug bites.

3) Imbalance: Rashes and Lumps

The following foods are recommended:

- Azuki bean strengthens the spleen and induces diuresis to reduce water retention. It clears heat and toxins and can even eliminate jaundice and boils (especially those that are caused by a damp-heat). Azuki beans are great for harmonizing the blood and can help to drain off pus. They can aid appendicitis, hemorrhoids, diarrhea, or dysentery with blood in stools. Eating azuki bean also helps to regulate blood, especially since stagnation of the blood can be responsible for many sensitivities.

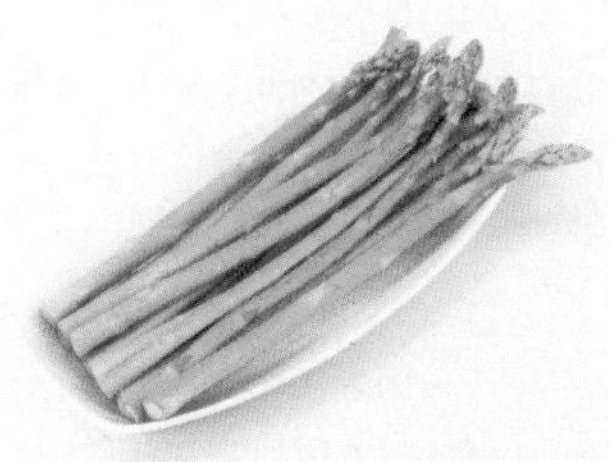
Fig. 76 Asparagus

- Asparagus (fig. 76) can be used to help treat dry skin and psoriasis. It is neutral and sweet in nature and enters the liver meridian. Asparagus helps to cool body heat and supports the production of body fluids, thereby also reducing thirst. Hepatitis and leucopenia can also be treated with asparagus.

External remedies:

- You may use a decoction of dandelion root leaf to apply on the skins surface.
- Add a little oil to the azuki bean powder (grind it fresh in a coffee grinder) and apply on the sensitive area of the skin or draining off skin pus. Keep it there for 30 minutes, then remove it.

Indigo Naturalis

In ancient time, it was dried and ground into a powder. This powder was painted onto the eyebrows to enhance their shape (fig. 77).

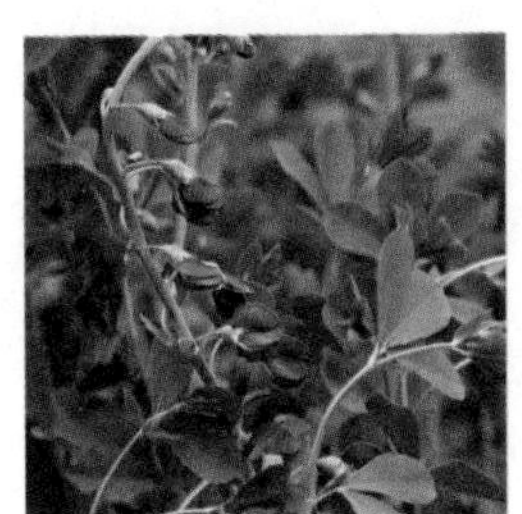
Fig. 77 Fresh indigo naturalis

In modern times this herb is used in herbal medicine for particular diseases and skin conditions. The taste is cold and salty and it is good for reducing inside heat. It is often used as a remedy for shingles, mumps, eczema and erysipelas (lymph infection in the head or legs). A very small quantity is used in preparations and should be prescribed by your TCM doctor.

4) Imbalance: Acne

One cause of acne may be eating too much meat in proportion to fruit and vegetables, or having too much heat in the lung. When too much lung heat causes acne, there may be more redness present in the pimples and on the face. Herbs to cool the lung and regulate the energy and movements in the upper portion of the body (upper energizer) can help to reduce or clear up face acne. Since the upper back and front of chest are also considered the lung section of the skin, noticing acne here can also sometimes be related to the lung.

The following foods are recommended:

- Mulberry leaf (fig. 78) and bark together with loquat fruit and leaf are powerful food sources to help solve the problem. If you cannot get access to the mulberry bark, then using the leaves in a tea is also beneficial.

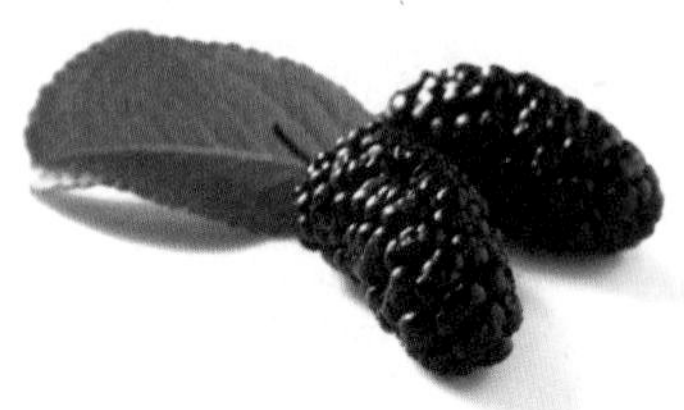

Fig. 78 Mulberry leaf and fruit

- Chamomile, dandelion and honeysuckle are also useful remedies. They may be taken together or separately. Usually, try them separately at first and then if the effect is not powerful enough, you can try to combine them. For the tea, you can use 3–6 g of dried leaves or flowers to make two to three cups of tea a day for a week.
- Those who have acne accompanied by damp heat, oily skin, and uneven skin tone could use pearl barley and mung beans in a soup. Use 30 g of pearl barley and 50 g of mung beans, soak them overnight to make them into a soup. Drink one cup twice a day, make sure you also eat 2 tsp of the barley and beans. Take this remedy for five

days.

- The cooling nature of watermelon is very effective for relieving toxic heat and can be used in spring and summer for those who develop acne or facial spider veins. Watermelon can also be used to ease a low-grade fever caused by high outdoor temperatures and humidity.

5) Imbalance: Warts

The following foods are recommended:

- Warts may be found on the body and can be treated by consuming a high dosage of pearl barley. Use 60 to 100 g for seven days in porridge or a soup. You might soak the pearl barley overnight and then add boiling water in the morning to stew for 30 minutes, and consume it as a tea.
- Warts on the hands and face (in a person with a damp constitution) can be treated by combining 60 g of pearl barley with 10 g of wood ear. Wash the wood ear, then soak for at least half an hour. Bring the ingredients to a boil, then simmer for 30 minutes. Eat this soup twice a day for ten days for maximum effectiveness.

External therapy:

- Rehydrate dried dark plums and smash them into a paste. Apply the paste to the area and leave it with a bandaid for at least 20 minutes and up to a few hours. Repeat this process and within a week warts may be removed.

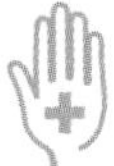

Pearl Barley Paste for Wrinkles

Wrinkles and stretch marks that appear after childbirth or weight loss can be combated with pearl powder and powdered pearl barley.

Use 60 g of powdered pearl barley and add 20 g of pearl powder, mixing thoroughly. Mix 2–5 g with oil or honey and make a thin paste. Apply to wrinkles and locally on the stretch marks once a day for a month.

6) Imbalance: Pigmentation

External remedy:

- The following Five-White Paste can help to decrease skin pigmentation. Empress Dowager Cixi, who was famous for her beautiful skin, used this recipe on her skin. She also used a angelica dahuricae (*bai zhi*) decoction to wash her face.

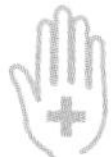

Treat Liver and Spleen for Pigmentation

In ancient times, it was common for people to use rose water to hydrate the skins surface. Rose water can be easily bough, but if you want to make your own, you can make it in a steamer. Place some fresh rose petals and mineral water in a bowl and steam for one hour. Put the liquid into a small container and spray it on your face.

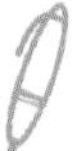

Other Functional Foods for Skin

Radix Cynanchi Auriculati (*bai shou wu*)

Radix Cynanchi Auriculati can be used both internally and externally for skin, hair, and breast beauty. It is neutral in temperature, slightly bitter, and sweet in taste. It enters the liver, kidney, spleen, and stomach channels. It is a tonic for the liver and kidney, strengthens tendon and bones, nourishes essence and blood, and strengthens spleen for digestion. It can also help to detoxify boils and malignant sores.

Angelica Dahuricae

Vitamin E oil mixed with powdered angelica dahuricae can be useful to heal scars. A note, some research has shown that it can make the skin a little more sensitive to the sun. So use it at night and be sure not to overexpose your skin to the sun when using it.

It is also very good to help excrete toxins in the blood, blood stagnation, and cysts. It is good for fungus, candida, and mold. You could drink ten pieces as a decoction for a short period of time. This herb is tolerated by most people, but it is always wise to work with your own TCM doctor who will prescribe according to your needs.

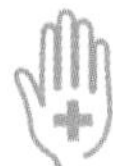

Five-White Paste

Ingredients: 6 g of angelica dahuricae, 6 g of Rhizoma Bletillae (*bai ji*), 6 g of poria, 5 g of chrysanthemum, 5 g of radix ampelopsis (*bai lian*)

How to Prepare?

1.Mix all the materials and grind them into a powder.

2.Mix the powder with some honey (optional coconut oil) and make a paste.

3.Put the paste on the pigmented area. Go to sleep and wash it off the next morning.

4.Continue for one month.

Healthy Nose

The nose is important as a tool for inhalation and interacting with the world through your sense of smell.

1) Imbalance: Sinus

A common problem that affects the nose is sinus blockages, which can enlarge the nose and leave you feeling generally uncomfortable.

External therapies:

- Bathing the nose with sea salt or using vinegar in a hot bowl of water to inhale the steam.
- Massaging down both sides of the nose starting at the eyebrows and finishing on either side of the nostrils. This may be repeated 20 times.
- Sniffing a lemon, mint (fig. 79), and citrus peel fragrance a few times a day can open nasal blockages.
- Breathing in smoke produced by burning dried corn silk is another remedy for treating chronic sinusitis.

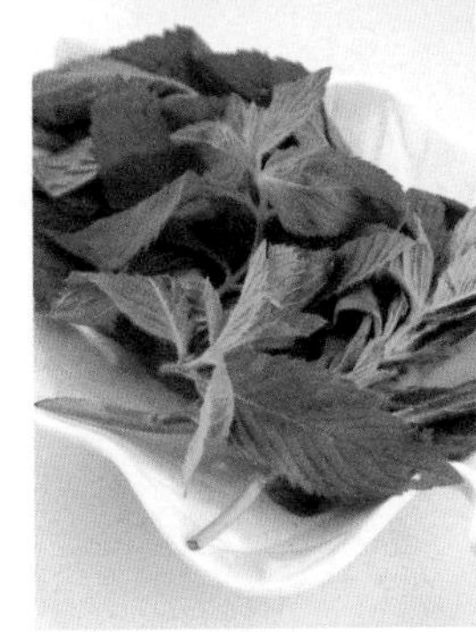

Fig. 79 Fresh mint

2) Imbalance: Running Nose

A constant runny nose can also be an inconvenient problem that leaves you feeling less than sexy. It can also contribute to broken skin around the nose from constant blowing, or a burning, dry sensation.

The following foods are recommended:

- Add spring onion to a delicious miso soup.
- Grape extract (fruit and seed) can be used as a food supplement for hay fever. It can help to combat itchy eyes, sneezing, and a running nose. Take two capsules once a day for two weeks.

External remedy:

- Use the white part of a spring onion (5 g) and make a tea ticture, which can be applied to the side of the nose.

3) Imbalance: Nosebleeds

A condition such as nosebleeds can occur when there is too much heat in the lung, or when a yin deficiency causes empty heat. Reducing the excess heat is an important step to reduce the occurrence of nosebleeds.

The following foods are recommended:

- Root of kalimeris indica (*ma lan*) is cool in temperature, spicy in taste, and enters the lung, liver, stomach and large intestine meridians. It expels the heat and cools the blood (fig. 80). It is also effectively deals with bleeding within the body and is likewise effective for nosebleeds. You can use it to make a tea.
- Raw winter melon juice is an effective recipe for nosebleeds. You could drink 120 ml twice a day

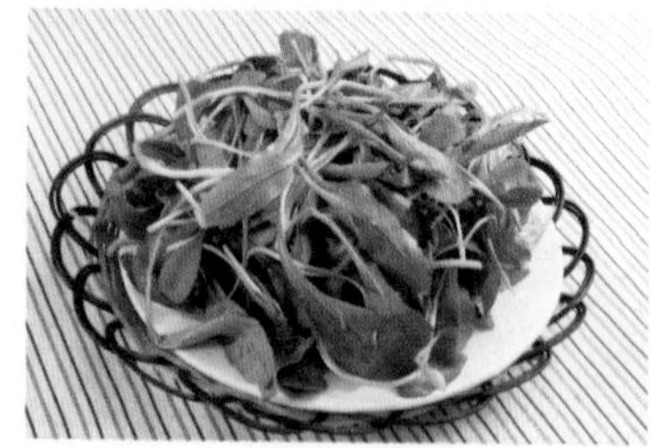

Fig. 80 Fresh kalimeris indica

for three days. It is slightly cold in temperature, sweet, and bland in taste and enters the lung, large and small intestines, and urinary bladder channels. Winter melon can induce diuresis, expel swelling, cool heat, produce body fluids and remove toxins. Externally apply the juice on effected area to treat nose boils and reduce rough nose skin pores.

4) Imbalance: Rosacea, Redness, and Swelling of the Nose

External therapy:

- Gingko nuts (two to three nuts) with gingko leaves (5 g) crushed into a paste can be very effective for dealing with rosacea and nose swelling. Once you have created a paste, rub it on the affected area and cover with a band aid, leave overnight. Remove to clean the nose and face the next morning. Repeat this every night for two weeks.

Fluid Metabolism

There are many conditions that can be helped by improving the metabolism of water in the upper body. The facial and cervical hydrologic cycle needs to be carefully nourished by the lung.

1) Imbalance: Puffy Face

A puffy face, especially around the cheek area and under the eyes, is caused by the inefficient flow of fluids in the head area. Since the lung help water flow from the eyes back to the nose and throat, then from the nose to the ears, a disruption in this pattern can be linked to the lung.

The water or lymph circulation in these areas may be disturbed after an invasion of cold or chronic sinus, or hay fever. Likewise, speeding up the lung's function of upper body water metabolism may treat a dripping feeling in the back of the throat and blocked ears. You could also work on the facial points to stimulate the different meridians of the Ren, large intestine and the stomach for the above-mentioned conditions.

External therapy:

- Gently massage the related points—Xiaguan point, Yingxiang point, and Tiantu point for improved fluid metabolism and to open blockages. Spend two to three minutes on each point massaging in small circles (fig. 81).

Fig. 81 The location of Xiaguan point, Yingxiang point, and Tiantu point

The following foods are recommended:

- Drink green tea for three days (3–5 g each day). A person with a very cold constitution could add a few drops of fresh ginger juice, since green tea is cooling in nature.
- You could use corn silk to make a soup or decoction for improving fluid metabolism in the upper body.

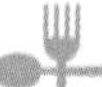

Silver Ear and Papaya Dessert

The following desert is delicious and can be used for anyone with combination facial skin (dry/oily) and to combat facial swelling (in those with mixed damp and dry constitutions).

Ingredients: 15 g silver ear, 1 papaya, crystal sugar (to taste)

How to Prepare?

1.Wash and soak silver ear for 30 minutes.

2.Cut papaya in half and remove seeds.

3.Boil the silver ear for 30 minutes (or use pre-cooked canned silver ear).

4.Add the crystal sugar to the silver ear, and put the mixture into the hollowed-out papaya halves.

5.Steam for 15 minutes.

6.Eat as dessert or snack three times a week for six weeks.

2) Imbalance: Hoarse Voice

The following foods are recommended:

- Momordica fruit (*luo han guo*) is sweet in taste and cool in temperature. It helps to clear lung heat, remove phlegm, and helps to remedy a dry, sore, and hoarse throat (fig. 82). Take 5 g and make a tea, and repeat for three days. In China, it is easy to find a candy made with momordica fruit to be used for these purposes.

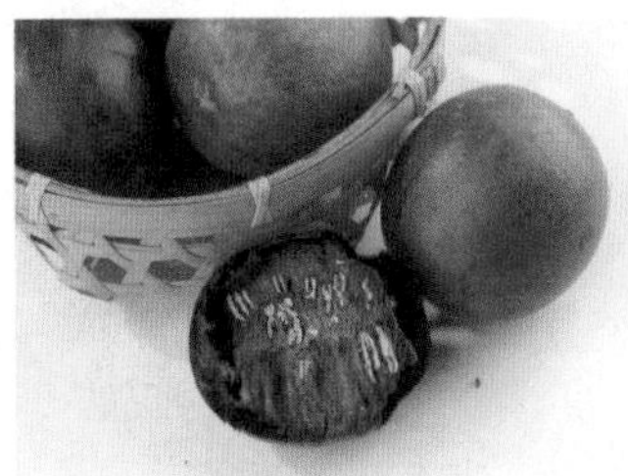

Fig. 82 Momordica fruits

- Fresh figs (or dried) can be eaten to help with a sore throat and hoarse voice. They can also help to remove mucus stagnation.
- Boat-fruited sterculia seed (*pang da hai*) is sweet and bland in taste and cool in temperature. It moistens the lung, sooths the throat, clear heat and also removes constipation. It is a lovely food supplements for teachers and singers. Use one piece in boiling water and place lid on it for five minutes. It will open up. Drink two to three cups per day by refilling the cup with boiling water, without adding more seeds. If you have diarrhea then this may not be the best option.

Your lung system bravely fights a constant battle to keep you and all your other organ systems healthy. It is the first line of defense in any invasion and is responsible for sending defensive qi to your skin's surface and nose. The lung plays a very important role in beautiful skin and ensures that the metabolism of fluids in your upper body are functioning smoothly. The oxygen and qi created by your lung is vital for your entire body. It is important to do everything you can to keep your lung system healthy.

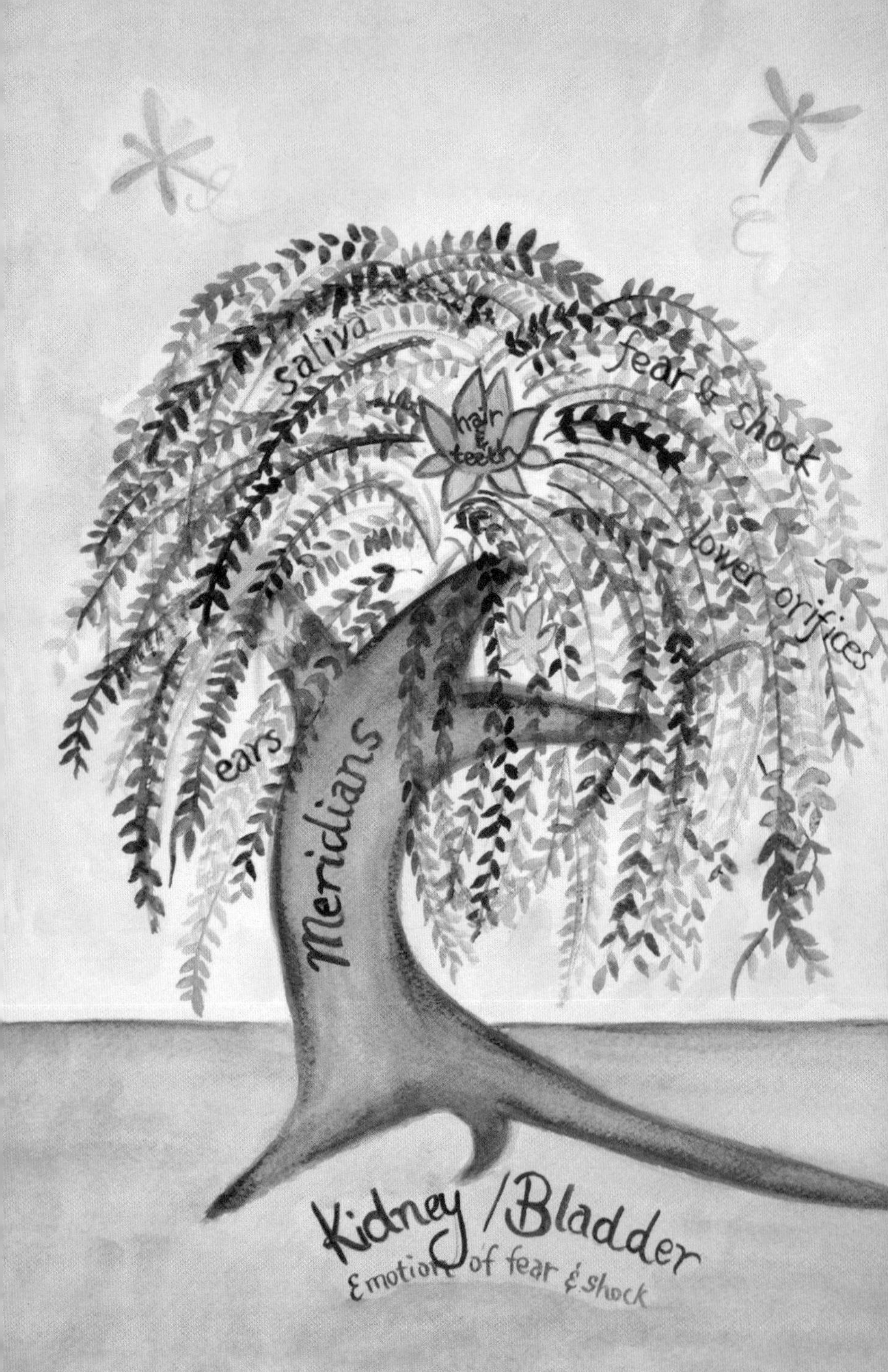
saliva
fear & shock
hair & teeth
lower orifices
ears
Meridians
Kidney / Bladder
Emotions of fear & shock

CHAPTER NINE
The Kidney System

Roots

- *Zang*-organ: kidney
- *Fu*-organ: urinary bladder
- Emotion of fear and shock

Trunk and Branches

- Meridians: Shaoyin Kidney Meridian of Foot, Taiyang Bladder Meridian of Foot

Leaves

- Well-structured bones
- Ears with keen hearing, which also control balance
- Timely self-eliminating lower orifices
- Thick saliva to nourish the mouth

Fruits

- Emotion of fear and shock (also part of the "roots" system)

Flowers

- Shiny, thick hair
- Beautiful white teeth

Left Fig. 83 The kidney system tree

1. Basic Facts about the Kidney System

You have two kidneys located in the back of your abdominal cavity. They are located quite low down close to your waist. The kidney and urinary bladder have a co-dependent relationship.

The kidney acts as the strength and intelligence of the entire body, and is responsible for its overall constitution. It is a storage facility for good essence. It governs the growth and development of the body as well as the maturation of the reproductive systems. It is the congenital base of life, and while partly based on heritage, one's own health management also influences the kidney's overall state.

The kidney is an important source of yin and yang can influence all the organ systems. The emotions linked to kidney are fear and fright. Kidney essence and qi help to build our structure and a fundamental base for the growth of bones, teeth, saliva, hearing, and healthy hair.

2. Functions of the Kidney

The kidney store both congenital and acquired essence, according to TCM.

All of the congenital essence you inherited from your ancestors and the accumulated essence you generate throughout your entire life will be stored in your kidney. Your kidney essence is not only for your own use, but also passed on to your children. This essence contributes to your DNA, but is not limited by this definition. It is like a bridge between generations past and generations to come. This in part explains the certain genetic markers that occur within family groups.

Many traditional cultures incorporate the use of special nourishing foods that women of childbearing age consume before pregnancy. In Chinese culture, kidney strength and health is highly valued. Before getting pregnant, a couple will often see a TCM doctor to make sure their kidney essence is robust. If any weakness is detected, then measures are taken to strengthen the kidney system. If a woman has difficulty getting pregnant, she may visit a TCM doctor who would check her kidney system.

It is not only the woman who pays special attention to her kidney essence. Men who experience loss of hair, ringing in the ears or weak hearing, and sore calf muscles (along the kidney meridian) may also visit a TCM doctor for treatment. Strengthening the kidney systems of the parents-to-be can give their child the best start in life. It is also fundamental to prevent early aging.

So what is kidney essence and why is it important?

Storing and Releasing Congenital and Acquired Essence

The first function of the kidney is the storage of essence. Essence can be transformed into qi to facilitate development and growth of your physical body, mental function, and reproductive system.

1) Types of Essence and the Basic Functions

There are two types of kidney essence. Both are stored in the kidney and mixed together to be used for your whole body:

- Congenital essence. It comes from your parents. It includes the genetic make-up required to program your physical appearance and genetic physiological features. This explains the commonalities between family members.
- Acquired essence. It can be created by eating nourishing food and through the inhalation of oxygen. Essence and qi can be transformed into each other, according to TCM. If you are short of qi, your body can use and transform some essence into it. Alternatively, if you have extra qi, your body can transform it into essence and store it in the kidney.

Congenital and acquired essence support and rely on each

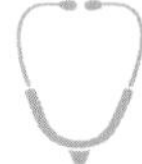

Reproductive System and Kidney Function

If your menstruation cycle is disturbed, and you are bleeding twice within the same month, and this persists over a long period of time, it can disrupt your kidney essence stores. People cannot produce blood quickly enough, and when this happens, your body will use your stored kidney essence.

The same is true as a result of too much ejaculation or in a situation where a man cannot control his seminal emission. Teenagers, when they are beginning to mature, might have some trouble in this area, but if an adult finds himself unable to control as he releases semen, then it might be caused by a weak kidney system.

other until a person reaches maturity. So kidney qi is acquired partly from congenital essence and partly from breathing and food.

The kidney is the root source of all the yin and yang in your body since it stores essence and qi. The essence belongs to yin and qi belongs to yang.

If people can tolerate summer heat well, then it is likely that their yin is sufficient. Those who can adjust to cold weather, less sun, and are able to work underground without feeling very uncomfortable, for instance, may have strong kidney.

In Chinese culture, the kidney also provides a timely release of essence through the process of menstruation and ejaculation. Your kidney is like a storehouse with their own time-release door. They have their own inbuilt function to control the release of essence. You might age more rapidly if the time-release door begins to allow too much essence to come out too quickly.

2) Facilitating the Body's Development and Growth

The kidney's role in storing and releasing kidney essence can ensure proper growth and development from infancy to old age.

It was described in the *Yellow Emperor's Canon* that there are various stages of growth and development. People can measure their own growth against the stages to ensure they were not burning through their essence too quickly.

You can certainly impact and slow down the rate of your aging through smart lifestyle choices. So you have the opportunity to create a life of balance to preserve your kidney essence.

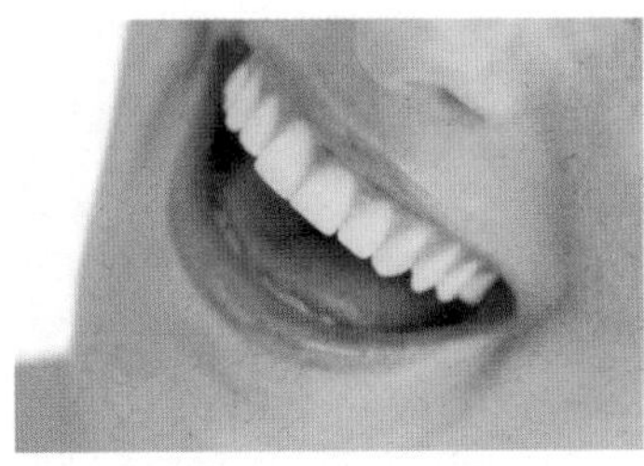

Fig. 84 Strong, firm, and white colored teeth make you look more youthful and they frame your smile.

It also provides a guideline for parents so that they can ensure their children are developing appropriately according to their age range. The developmental stages go up in increments of seven for females and eight for males. During childhood, kidney essence is responsible for the proper growth of bones, teeth, hair, and the brain.

For instance, a 14-year-old who has developed some white hair is demonstrating a tell-tale sign of weak kidney essence. A TCM doctor might address this by prescribing food remedies, herbs, or acupuncture.

Baby teeth are exchanged for adult teeth at approximately age seven for girls and age eight for boys, according to the *Yellow Emperor's Canon*. Growth of the physical body and cognitive learning is rapid. Weak kidney essence might be observed in children who have poor bone growth or teeth development (fig. 84). Some learning difficulties can also be traced back to kidney essence imbalances.

At approximately age 14 for girls and 16 for boys, reproductive hormones are formed and the related meridians open up. This enables young women to begin a regular menstrual cycle, and for males to be able to ejaculate. During puberty, both sexes begin to have the ability to conceive.

Menstrual issues during this time can sometimes be traced

back to the kidney, such as delayed or early menstruation.

Early menstruation has become a common occurrence amongst young girls in modern times. Some girls are beginning menstruation from as early as 8-year-old. This in part is due to hormones that are added to our food sources. Most people are aware of factory farming which uses growth hormones to raise animals quickly. A chicken that traditionally took one year and a half to grow can now be raised in three months and ready for consumption. Furthermore, it is believed by some, that monitoring what your young ladies watch on television is also important to avoid early menstruation. Many modern movies contain fairly explicit sexual content and this content may be responsible for stimulating hormones to develop before their time.

In fact, there are many TCM hospitals in China that offer treatment protocols to delay menstruation for a few years for young girls who begin menstruating too early. This helps to preserve their kidney essence and help it reach its full potential before it begins to periodically release during regular menstrual cycles. Normal breast development may begin from 8–12 years old and menstruation might begin anywhere from 11 to 14 years of age. Anything outside this range might need addressing.

On the other side of the spectrum, if a boy reaches the age of 16 and his voice hasn't changed or Adam's apple hasn't developed, and he has not begun to ejaculate; or a girl has not begun to regularly menstruate, strengthening kidney essence might be a useful strategy.

It is important that kidney essence is stored up to the age of about 12 to 14 for girls and about 14 to 16 for boys. If it leaks out earlier than this, then it may never reach its full potential.

Young adulthood begins at age 21 for females and 24 for males. During this time, kidney energy is even and robust. Wisdom teeth start to grow and hair is full and thick.

The next phase of growth, according to the *Yellow Emperors*

Canon, occurs at age 28 for young women and 32 for men. During this time, the mind has a good ability to innovate, the physical body is harmonized, hair reaches its longest growth potential, and the physical structures of the body are strong and resilient. The spine, muscles, tendons, ligaments, and bones are at their best. Issues with conception or chronic miscarriages might be caused by weak kidney essence and qi during this age bracket.

When women reach age 35 and men the age of 40, the "yangming" category meridian starts to slowdown in growth. Not as much energy reaches your face and for women especially, this may result in the appearance of fine lines and some wrinkles. Men are more vulnerable to the loss of teeth during this phase of development. Hair loss may also begin to become apparent. For women, issues with conception or miscarriage may be traced back to the kidney during these years. It is thought that if you have really long thick hair in your thirties, forties, and fifties you might have very strong kidney essence.

There is somewhat of a natural decline of the physical body after the ages of 42 for women and 48 for men. Of course, being aware of this fact can help us make wise choices to encourage anti-aging and preservation of our health and appearance. Conservation of kidney essence becomes a useful strategy and this can be encouraged in part by developing habits of moderation in diet, exercise, sexual activity, and life balance.

Kidney essence stores may also be added to by developing positive breathing habits, and with activities such as *tai ji* and *qi gong*. During this phase of life, the three yang categories of

The "Yangming" Category Meridians

These meridians start to slowdown in growth after women reach age 35 and men the age of 40.

- Yangming Large Intestine Meridian of Hand
- Yangming Stomach Meridian of Foot

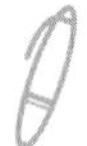

Three Yang Categories of Meridians

These meridians will become a little weaker in the upper portion of the body after the ages of 42 for women and 48 for men.

- Taiyang Bladder Meridian of Foot
- Taiyang Small Intestine Meridian of Hand
- Yangming Large Intestine Meridian of Hand
- Yangming Stomach Meridian of Foot
- Shaoyang Gallbladder Meridian of Foot
- Shaoyang *San jiao* Meridian of Hand

meridians all become a little weaker in the upper portion of the body and additional fine lines and wrinkles might start to appear along with grey hair. Men might start to experience some more grey hairs on their sideburns.

At approximately age 49 for women and 56 for men, there are further changes in the physical body.

For women, the special meridian linked to the reproductive system, including the ovaries and uterus have less energy flow. The reproductive hormones decrease tremendously resulting in the inability to conceive for some women. Changes in your body weight might also occur including some additional weight around the mid-section or muscle atrophy. Some height loss might also occur due to bone loss.

Liver energy for the men begins to weaken, tendons might become less flexible, and reproductive hormones also decrease. The storage of kidney essence lowers and the physical body may become weaker.

It is vital that from this period onwards, you do all that you can to conserve your kidney essence stores to avoid rapid aging. Working for three days in a row with no sleep might have been possible when you were younger. In your older years, this will cause you to burn through your kidney essence too quickly if you maintain this type of lifestyle.

As can be seen from the description of aging in the *Yellow Emperors Canon*, the kidney plays a very important role in beauty. Any kind of condition linked to the teeth, hair, sexual activity, and reproductive system are all linked back to kidney essence and qi; and a balance of yin and yang. An upright posture is also a sign of strong kidney essence that is nourishing the bones and spine. Preserving both congenital and acquired essence, and using them as slowly as possible is an effective anti-aging strategy. Adding to these stores through positive lifestyle choices is also important.

3) Creating Yin-Yang Balance

All the yin and yang in your body is created in the kidney and then distributed to the organs. This yin and yang comes from kidney essence and qi. As you can imagine, balanced yin and yang is important for your whole body system especially for the balance between cold and heat in your body.

Deficiency of kidney yang can influence spleen and heart yang, and ultimately lead to different weaknesses within the body related to these conditions. Symptoms such as cold limbs and hands, muddy thinking, confusion, inadequate mental energy, and cold pain in the waist area can all be linked to kidney yang weakness. Having inadequate kidney yang also does not lead to a strong spirit. Other symptoms might include: knee weakness, the inability to stand for long periods of time, very clear and large quantities of urine, edema, and early morning diarrhea. Some of these symptoms come from a spleen or heart imbalance, but have their root cause in kidney weakness. Therefore, it becomes necessary to address the kidney as the root of the problem.

Kidney yin deficiency will manifest with a different set of symptoms. Some of these include a five palm heat (soles of the feet, palms and chest), hot flushes, night sweats, dizziness, tinnitus (ringing in the ears), a dull ache, and weakness in the lower back and knees. Men may struggle with controlling seminal emission. This may occur when watching a movie or in the form of a wet dream, but the root cause may be kidney yin deficiency.

For kidney yang and yin deficiencies, it is important to support and tonify the kidney essence and qi to rebalance it. Just tonifying yin and yang may not be enough. So in a case where someone has low yin, it may be recommended that they strengthen their yin by consuming some yin forming foods and/or herbs as well as strengthening their kidney essence and qi.

Governing Water Metabolism

The kidney is known as the water organ, according to Five Elements Theory. It receives body fluids from the lung, then metabolizes good body fluids, and directs wastewater to the urinary bladder for elimination. These functions are dependent upon kidney qi.

1) Reusing Body Fluid and Dispelling Waste

The Kidney has the ability to identify how much body fluid the body needs and to transform it so that it can be used again. It is also important for the kidney to be able to recognize which fluid to eliminate.

The opening where urine is expelled is like a door, when and how wide this door opens is dependent upon the kidney, according to TCM. If the door is constantly opening or doesn't open enough, then TCM will treat the kidney system. Before you treat kidney disharmony, you should also check that you are not going overboard with your water consumption.

Problems with the inability to pass urine and on the other end of the spectrum, incontinence are linked back to a weak kidney system. And treating the kidney can also help people with the following situations:

- If you are unable to pass urine or control the passing of your urine, this can really impact your body and upset your whole body's water balance. You should pass urine approximately 6–8 times a day.

- If you have to go to the bathroom every half an hour or need to go more than three times during the night, then it would be prudent to address kidney function. Passing urine more than three times a night may indicate a disturbance of your yang energy. Of course, pregnancy and old age are exceptions.
- Older children who experience bedwetting.
- Men who experience prostate problems with issues of frequent urine.
- Water retention below the waist, lower back pain, or knee pain can all be signs that your kidney might need rebalancing.

Tips for lifestyle:

- Water is useful for detoxifying, but should not be overdone. Overdoing plain water can weaken your yang qi. Liquid that comes from food and soups contain many minerals. Drinking a lot of distilled water is not very good for the body as it is devoid of minerals. We are often told to drink a lot of water, but drinking too much can be problematic, too. Your water needs are dependent upon how much you sweat, how much exercise you do, how hot it is, and whether you are talking a lot. All these factors will increase your water needs.
- In China, older people always drink warm water even in the summer, and they are very careful to keep their ice-cream consumption down to a very small quantity.
- Be aware of seasonal changes. During winter when you don't sweat much, you might need to reduce your water intake. You should be able to wait two and a half hours in-between toilet visits. So if you are going every half an hour, you should ensure that you do not have any underlying conditions.

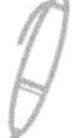

Chinese Life Style

In the Chinese way of thinking, water isn't any kind of tonic, so liquids that add nutrition or nourishment are favored. Chinese people favor soups and nourishing teas over plain water.

- They get water from fruit, porridge, and other sources. They take into account their activity levels, job, and individual constitution.
- When the weather is cold, having soup three times a day before meals as well as some nourishing tea, and a few glasses of water throughout the day is enough for most people.
- During the summer, Chinese people consume more watermelon and some raw vegetables, which also contain water and contribute to body fluids.

In the West, people drink less soup so this should also be taken into consideration.

2) Promoting Water Metabolism for Other Organs

In addition to its job of filtering your body's water and sending wastewater to the urinary bladder for elimination, your kidney also influences the water metabolism of the other organs.

It directly influences spleen yang and lung qi due to the fact that spleen and lung are supported by kidney yin and yang.

Supported by adequate kidney yin and yang, the spleen can absorb liquid food to produce body fluids. The spleen then sends body fluids to the lung and also the limbs and muscles.

The lung's ascending and descending functions are also dependent upon help from a well-functioning kidney. Through its ascending and descending mechanisms, body fluids will be distributed to every part of the body.

3) Governing the Reception of Qi

The kidney can govern the reception of qi and receive lung qi. The lung is the governing organ of qi, and the kidney is the root organ of qi, according to TCM. The kidney plays a role in storing and holding qi from the upper portion of the body to the lower portion of the body.

When the lung takes in oxygen, the body needs to cooperate with the kidney in order to create deeper breathing. When you inhale, kidney energy comes up and attempts to meet the lung's energy. Once this happens, the kidney energy pulls the qi down and draws it into itself. If you breathe deeply, the kidney will more likely be successful in bringing this energy down.

During meditation, people often breathe in through the nose and then hold the breath for a few seconds, holding the breath in will help the kidney perform this duty of pulling qi down from the lung into the *dan tian* area (below the belly button).

We can liken kidney qi to a receptionist of a company. Just as a receptionist will come out to meet the visitors and guide them to their destination, the kidney qi performs the very important duty of pulling lung qi down and guiding it to the *dan tian*.

When this process is completed successfully, original qi and acquired qi become harmonized and your storage of qi will be of a high quantity. This is why many restorative exercises focus on breathing as a means to restore the body's energy levels. By doing this regularly, your ability to hold qi will be enhanced, and you will not easily loose or waste it.

If you immediately feel short of breath as a result of walking, climbing up stairs, or when walking uphill, for example, it may be assumed that your kidney is not receiving qi from the lung. This

Ways of Meditation

By doing this meditation you will create more qi for the same quantity of oxygen.

Step 1: Breathe in as deeply as you can through your nose.

Step 2: Hold the breath for 20 seconds, then breathe out slowly through your mouth.

Step 3: Do this for a few minutes for renewed energy and for qi accumulation.

function of the kidney helps to facilitate deeper breathing, quality breaths, and allows us to store a little bit of extra qi.

Swimmers and long distance runners may be unwittingly developing this skill, because as your lung expands the kidney energy will find it easier to come up and meet lung qi. You may have noticed that when you first begin a fitness regime, you may find yourself short of breath very quickly. After a few months of training, you may begin to find it easier to complete the same tasks. Enhancing fitness trains breathing and training breathing can enhance fitness. Over time, your kidney will become more skilled at drawing lung qi into the *dan tian* and this will help you not feel tired as quickly.

3. Meridians of the Kidney System

The Shaoyin Kidney Meridian of Foot starts under the 5th toe, and runs to the base of the foot, travels up behind the ankle, on the inside of the leg up to the inner aspect of the thigh. It then comes up towards the sacrum, it ascends along the lumbar spine, and enters the kidney and urinary bladder. From there, it travels into the abdominal region, passes through the diaphragm, and enters the chest. It then ascends to the throat and terminates at the root of the tongue (fig. 85).

The Taiyang Bladder Meridian of Foot begins in the inside corner of the eye goes through the forehead, over the top of the head down to the nape of the neck, and travels in two lines on each side of the spine. From the lumbar area, it enters the kidney and bladder. It then travels over the glutes and down the back of the legs past the hamstrings, calves, outside of the ankles and feet, and ends at the little toe (fig. 86).

The kidney and bladder have a co-dependent relationship in two areas. Firstly, they work together to produce urine, and

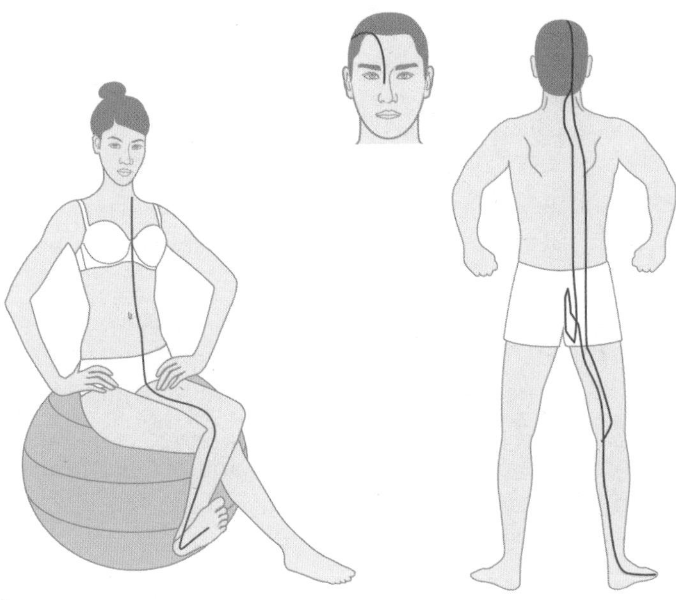

Fig. 85 Shaoyin Kidney Meridian of Foot

Fig. 86 Taiyang Bladder Meridian of Foot

secondly they cooperate with each other through meridians and points to excrete urine.

The kidney is the water metabolism organ. All the waste from the body's fluids will eventually travel to the kidney and from the kidney to the urinary bladder. The urinary bladder may store urine for awhile before excreting it. Once enough urine has accumulated the kidney's transforming energy is vital to let the urine out.

Pathologically, damp heat from the urinary bladder can invade the kidney, according to TCM. In Western medicine, we might describe this condition as a urinary bladder infection that has led to a secondary kidney infection. Symptoms might present such as painful, yellow urine with a burning sensation as

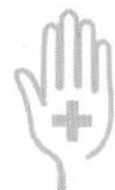

Use a Jade *Gua Sha* Board

Using a jade *gua sha* board (jade enters into the heart and lung meridians), gently move it on your face, repeat 20 times. It is really effective to prevent winkles and sagging skin.

it is excreted, an urgency to go but then only small amounts of urine coming out; and a sensation of the urinary channel being blocked.

In a severe cases, kidney stones may form, since a damp heat is the perfect condition for stones and polyps to grow. In this case, you might strengthen the kidney and treat the damp heat in the urinary bladder.

Many yang surfaces of the body belong to the urinary bladder channels. The back of your body is the yang surface as well as the top of the head. Although there are not many herbs used for the urinary bladder, there are many manual treatments that can benefit this system including acupuncture, cupping, *tui na*, and *gua sha*.

4. Kidney System and Beauty

The kidney controls your body's essence, then your essence contributes to your body's "marrow". In TCM, "marrow" does not just refer to bone marrow like in Western medicine. Rather, it refers to the common matrix of the three types of marrow found in your body: bone marrow, brain marrow, and spinal cord matter.

Bones: Tissue of the Kidney

In TCM, the three types of marrow are all produced as a result of kidney essence. The marrow has its own special blood circulation to ensure that the bones receive enough nutrition.

Any kind of bone disorder, such as brittleness has a strong connection to the kidney.

Likewise, strong healthy bones are formed as a result of a strong kidney system and those with robust kidney will be able to stand for long periods of time and complete hard work without tiring easily. Those who cannot stand for longer than ½ hour and those who cannot commit to hard work may have a kidney imbalance.

There are many signs that communicate to us that the kidney may need extra love:

- In infancy, the hole on the top of a baby's skull should close within the first two years. If it is late closing, is weakly closed, or doesn't close flat then it may indicate that the bones haven't received enough essence from the marrow.
- Issues with teeth (which are the outward manifestation of your bones) can also flag warning signs that the kidney needs balancing. Some people's baby teeth are very slow in changing to adult teeth and in certain cases don't occur until adulthood. The appropriate age for this to happen is between the ages of 7–12 years old. Many families in ancient China used to collect each baby tooth lost to ensure that all the teeth had fallen out and were replaced by adult teeth. The kidney would be treated if this was not the case.
- The condition whereby a child has soft bones and is still unable to walk at the age of six can also be treated by working on the kidney and kidney essence.
- In adulthood, osteoporosis, weak soft knees, back pain when standing for long periods of time, and teeth that break easily are signs of diminished kidney essence.
- Losing your teeth too early, for instance during menopause, or in your 30's and 40's may indicate that

your kidney essence is insufficient.

- Elderly people who easily fracture bones and are uncoordinated when walking may need to support their kidney essence. In modern times, we attribute these conditions, in part, to the lack of calcium. In addition to including more calcium in the diet, it is also prudent to tonify the kidney. Just adding calcium supplements is not enough and some studies have indicated that calcium supplements may not be absorbed well and may end up accumulating in the arteries. Tonifying the kidney can help you more effectively store calcium from your food into your bones. In China, the use of food rather than pills has been a popular course of action. Bone soups, dried small shrimp, soup, and soymilk are all used to add to dietary calcium.
- Spine and brain marrow are very important for hearing, vision, and good mental capacities. The ability to adapt, react with fast responses, and to think quickly are all based on spine and brain marrow. In TCM, the material of the brain is more related to the kidney, and the mental function of the brain is more related to the heart. If the spine and brain marrow become deficient due to weak kidney essence, people may experience symptoms of dull thinking, slow response, blurred vision, deafness, ringing in the ears, and mental fatigue (the body seems ok, but the mind easily tires). All of these symptoms may be related to a deficiency of the spine and brain marrow. In the worst case scenario, early onset of Alzheimer's may occur.

Ears: Window of the Kidney

The kidney supports the function of hearing and the balance control centers found in your ears.

Brain marrow is especially important for these functions.

If a person has sufficient brain marrow, they will have sensitive hearing.

In China, hearing problems and early stage tinnitus are often treated by addressing the kidney meridians or by using kidney herbs or food tonics. The earlier treatment is received the better. If someone has completely lost their hearing, then tonifying the kidney may not help. It is important to get in and treat these symptoms early. Some children are born with poor hearing and getting them to a good TCM treatment program quickly may help improve this condition.

Lower Orifices: A Link to the Kidney

Women have three lower orifices. They have a channel to eliminate urine, the vagina, and an anus. Men have two, an anus and a single channel that both excretes urine and also seminal fluids.

The excretion of urine is controlled by the urinary bladder, but the kidney supports this function. Anyone suffering with urinary bladder problems may also need to address their kidney system. Clinically, there are more methods to help the kidney than the urinary bladder.

The vagina and the penis are also related to the reproductive system. So a clear connection can be drawn between them and the kidney system.

The anus's function is to excrete stools, and therefore, it is more related to the large intestine, spleen, and stomach. However, there are some cases, such as early morning diarrhea that may be clinically connected to the kidney. Constipation or the inability to control stool elimination, particularly in older people, and some cases of diarrhea may require a kidney tonic.

Thick Saliva: Controlled by the Kidney

The kidney controls the thick saliva in the mouth that is

produced under the tongue. When you relax or meditate, your body produces a little bit more of this type of saliva, and it is better to swallow it rather than spit it out.

When you do *tai ji,* it is important to place the tip of the tongue on the roof of your mouth. As you breathe throughout the movements, your body will automatically produce more of this type of saliva. You should swallow it afterwards. This thick saliva when swallowed has similar benefits to eating edible bird's nest.

Edible bird's nest is a popular beauty food eaten in Asia, renowned for producing beautiful skin. This type of saliva nourishes kidney essence. During sexual activity when you are kissing your partner, you will also produce this kind of saliva as your tongues touch. It is believed that if you swallow this saliva, it will enrich your kidney essence.

Hair: Flower of Kidney

Hair is the flower of the kidney. Gorgeous hair can be a reflection of strong kidney essence.

Hair growth needs a lot of blood. It is actually considered to be the "left over of your body's blood", according to TCM. This is why you lose hair when you have anemia conditions, other conditions where you have insufficient blood, or are receiving chemotherapy. Hair also needs kidney essence. If you have a blood deficiency, you might find it difficult to grow your hair.

Thinning hair or insufficient hair growth can indicate that kidney function is getting weaker and a lot can be done to stop excess hair loss as you age. The color, growth of your hair is dependent upon the kidney, and the shininess and moisture of the hair is dependent upon the blood. If your body does not have enough blood, then it will prioritize the organs and your hair will suffer. Remember, essence and blood have a special relationship. If you have a lot of blood left over, it can transfer back into essence so you never need to worry about having too much blood. If at any particular time you don't have enough blood, then your essence stores will be used to convert into blood ultimately leading to diminished essence.

Strengthening kidney essence and tonifying blood can help any sort of hair loss, dry or grey hair, and split ends. Grey hair is often seen as hereditary because you inherit your congenital kidney essence from your parents, but you can really tonify the kidney to delay the aging process.

Mental jobs can consume a lot of brain marrow so very stressful mental jobs may rob your hair from nourishment if you do not take measures to nourish your kidney. If you take action, you can slow down or even stop the hair loss. When you first notice some grey hairs, you might seek to strengthen the kidney through Chinese medicine and delay more from appearing.

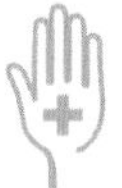

Massage for Thick Eyebrows and Eyelashes

Castor oil can be used to help thicken eyebrows and eyelashes. It is high in many minerals and helps them grow. Use a small brush or cotton bud to apply the oil in the areas where you would like to see more growth. Let it absorb as you massage it in. You should notice a little redness as you stimulate blood flow to the area. When massaging the eyebrows, you are also massaging some gallbladder and *san jiao* points so you are getting the added benefit of regulating the gallbladder and *san jiao*.

Fear and Fright: Emotions of the Kidney

The emotions associated with the kidney are fear and fright.

Fear is the same as worry and some people are more susceptible to fears than others. Fear could be based in reality or on a phobia. For instance, you might feel afraid if a tiger is chasing you, or have a fear of heights, claustrophobia, or a fear of spiders.

Shock or fright can occur as a result of certain events. For instance, you may be travelling in an airplane that experiences mechanical problem and may fall from the sky for several meters. In this case, you would experience a sudden fright, but would hopefully recover from it quite quickly.

Fright and fear are both related to kidney balance and strength. Those with a strong kidney system might have a high tolerance to fear and shock, and may not be rattled easily.

On the other hand, long term or chronic fear may cause injury to kidney qi and cause it to sink down. Eventually, the sinking of kidney qi might lead to involuntary urine, stool, or seminal emission.

We have heard of occurrences where someone has experienced an extreme fright and has had an uncontrolled bowel motion or "wet themselves", even animals in the wild when they are frightened often have a bowel movement. Kidney essence that is constantly sinking down due to these extreme or chronic emotions may not be able to rise up to collect lung qi. This affects kidney essence production and leads to a vicious cycle of low kidney qi.

It is very important to transform feelings of fear and phobia. You may have had a big shock if you were caught in an earthquake or escaped an erupting volcano. If you do not deal with the fear and allow it to turn into a long-term phobia, you may drain your kidney qi and essence over the long term.

Furthermore, in China it is believed that pregnant women should be careful about watching horror films or films that cause a reaction of shock because it could be injurious to the kidney or in an extreme case, may lead to a miscarriage.

5. Beauty Problems and Enhancement

Now we will discuss three beauty concerns that are related to your kidney system and will provide some acupressure points, massage methods, food options, and herbal recipes that will benefit this system.

If however, you cannot seem to rebalance your kidney system and relieve your symptoms using the natural and herbal remedies provided, you might seek treatment by seeing a TCM doctor who can help strengthen qi, restore yin-yang balance, and harmonious organ systems.

The color black and the salty taste corresponds with the kidney. Black foods are best for winter, a season when, according to TCM, one should store energy. The kidney system plays a role in this, and black foods promote and strengthen the kidney system. Research shows that most black foods are rich in inorganic salt and melanin.

Heavenly Hair

Hair is often described as your crowning glory. We all have different colored hair. However, healthy hair will be thick, easy to grow, shiny, smooth, soft, and elastic. We loose and grow approximately 50 to 100 new hairs each day. How much hair we have may be dependent upon the health of the hair follicles and genetic factors.

This section of the book is dedicated to the topics of hair loss, balding in patches, and grey or white hair. As already mentioned, healthy hair is dependent upon a healthy kidney system and well-nourished kidney essence. Both kidney yin and yang deficiency can cause all of the above-mentioned conditions. TCM would address these issues internally and externally. Furthermore, since the hair is "the leftover of the blood", when blood becomes deficient, too hot, or stagnated, it may affect certain areas of the scalp. This can cause a lack of thickness or slow growth of hair in certain regions.

Yin and yang deficiencies can impact your hair and scalp.

Yin deficiency is a deficiency of body fluids, blood and essence. Yang deficiency causes a disruption of the smooth movements of qi and efficient flow of qi in the meridians.

If you want glorious hair, it is important to nourish the yin and yang in your body. In fact, the head is the crossroads for many of the yang meridians. It is common to use a yang tonic and at the same time stimulate the meridians and flow of qi on the head area for hair and scalp conditions.

Severe emotionally traumatic experiences could be a cause for sudden greying or hair loss. In this case, the liver may send too much liver heat and fire to the head area, causing an over consumption of body fluids and blood. There have been extreme cases of where greying has literally occurred within a few days or over a very short period of time.

Kidney yang deficiency could manifest as an aversion to cold or wind, especially in the head, hands, and feet. It could also present as a cold feeling in the body or even deep into the organs that you just can't shake.

There are many food sources and herbs that can be used effectively as kidney yin or yang tonics and some great ones that help to regulate liver heat.

The following foods are recommended for regulating kidney yin:

Eating a lot of black sesame seeds, walnuts, and supplementing with some fo-ti root can be very helpful for re-growing nice strong hair. The remedies mentioned below are also good for the blood and can support the mental and physical needs of the body so that there is enough blood left over for beautiful hair. You could make a nut milk using walnuts, sesame seeds (fig. 87), and honey. You could consume this warm or at room temperature. You may alternatively add a teaspoon of ground walnut and sesame seed powder to the top of your rice two to three times per week. This is also very easy to make and it is best to make it fresh and consume it quickly so that the oils do not become rancid. Actually, nuts and seeds are recommended for consumption only when they are in season.

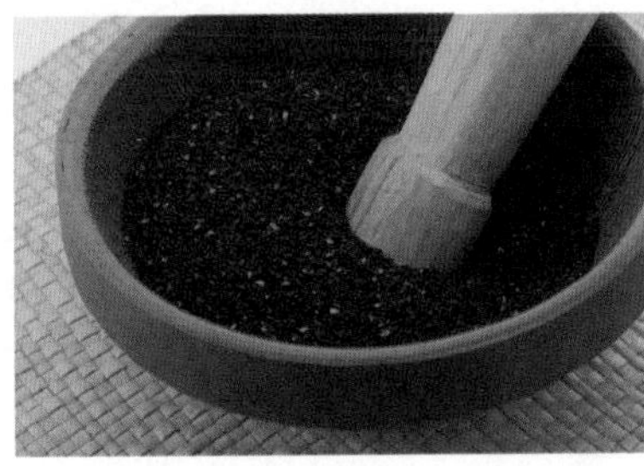
Fig. 87 Black sesame seeds

- Fo-ti root is held in high esteem in China and is a powerful blood tonic. Many Chinese women, as they age, use multiple strategies to remain youthful, such as modifying their diet so that they can remain the same weight as when they first married and using herbs such as fo-ti root to maintain strong, thick black hair with a deep rich color. It should not, however, be taken on a continuous basis without a break. And when used in the context mentioned above, it may be taken for only one or two months per year in tablet or root form. If using the root, it can be added to soup. Some people make it into a tea. Many women in China, between the ages of 48–50 take two cups in the afternoon. It can also be used to combat constipation, nourish the brain, and is well known for delaying grey hairs once they start to appear.
- Fresh and dried mulberries nourish yin and increase blood. Mulberry fruit prevents and treats dizziness, tinnitus, premature grey hair, and weakness in the lower back. They are enriching to the body fluid and help moisturize dryness. Mulberries also prevent and treat dry stools and rapid hair loss. They can also boost the immune system and increase blood count.

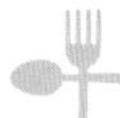

Treat Spleen for Heavenly Hair

Wood ear is good for strengthening qi and nourishing blood. Low qi is characterized by mental and physical fatigue. Those who are pale in the face and lips, or who have a yellow complexion suffer from a deficiency of blood. It is effective for those who have prematurely aged with grey hair.

Women should pay extra attention to boosting their blood by consuming blood tonics since they lose a large amount each month through menstruation. Wolfberries, jujubes, and red kidney beans are great for this purpose. In fact, many foods that are red in color are good for the blood and any food that is black in color is great for the kidney.

The following foods are recommended for regulating kidney yang. Warming foods and spices are good for kidney yang. The below ones are great inclusions:

- Dried ginger warms the lung, kidney, and digestive system. Furthermore, it strengthens yang and facilitates circulation. It is a powerful tonic for painful joints, and heavy and numb feelings in the four limbs.
- Sword beans can tonify and warm the kidney and stimulate yang. They can also be used to reduce aches in the sides of the abdomen and can treat hernia and lumbago.
- Raspberry is a liver, kidney, and yang tonic.
- Walnuts (fig. 88) strengthen the kidney and warm the lung: As a medicine, walnuts are used for asthma and coughs, including symptoms of chronic coughing, wheezing with shortness of breath, clear or white watery mucus, and exercise-induced asthma. These conditions are common in people who have an aversion to cold during seasonal changes, especially children and the elderly. They also treat weaknesses, such as those with

weaknesses in the back or bladder. Furthermore, knee pain, problems with seminal emission, or urinary incontinence can be helped by eating walnuts.

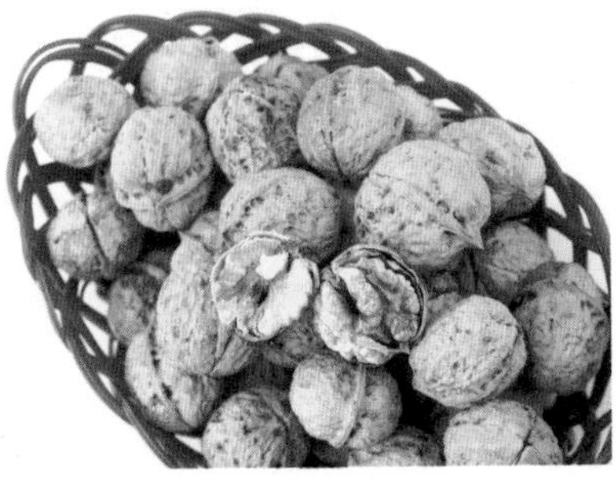

Fig. 88 Walnuts

- Chai tea (which may include clove, fennel, cinnamon, and black tea) can help to warm the body and tonify the yang.
- Cinnamon bark is hot in nature and is good for strengthening kidney yang and increasing vitality. In this case, those who would benefit from cinnamon usually suffer from lower back pain or cold in that region as well as the frequent need to urinate with little flow. Other signs specifically for men may be the tendency toward impotency or nocturnal emission, while women may have amenorrhea or show signs of infertility. Children over three years old who are still wetting the bed may also benefit from including cinnamon in the diet.

External Remedies:

- You may use either rosemary water or ginger juice in the areas where there is insufficient hair growth. Ginger could be a particularly good choice for those with oily hair and rosemary might be more appropriate for dry or normal hair. Ginger juice can be made very quickly by grating the ginger and straining the juice. Alternatively, you could cook either the ginger or rosemary in water, then strain, and use the liquid on areas of your scalp where you would like to stimulate hair growth.
- Vinegar might be good to use when the liver is

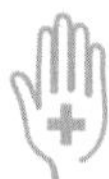

Apply a Hair Massage

1.Using your fingers or wooden comb, begin combing your hair from the front to the back of your head. Cover the entire scalp.

2.Then begin to massage your scalp with your fingertips, with light pressure, using small circular motions (clockwise then anti-clockwise 20 times each).

3.At the Baihui point, spend a little bit of extra time because this is the junction where all the yang energy meridians pass across each other (fig. 89). Baihui literally means "hundred junction", and is a powerful meeting point of many meridians in your body. Concentrating on this point can help increase the yang energy in your organs and create more energy in your body. It can also draw circulation to your scalp.

Baihui point (DU 20)

Top of the head

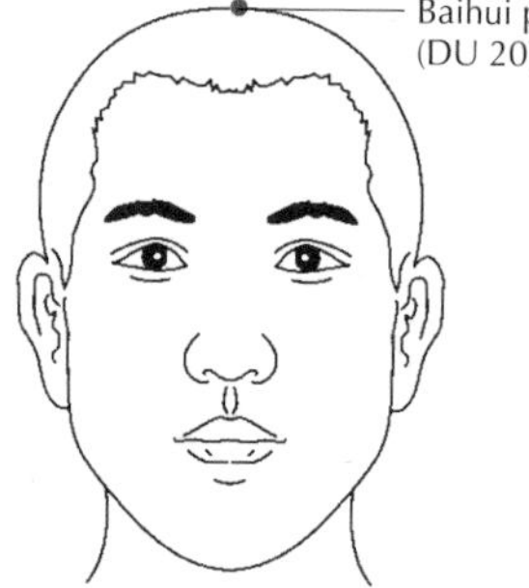

Front of the head

Fig. 89 Location of Baihui point

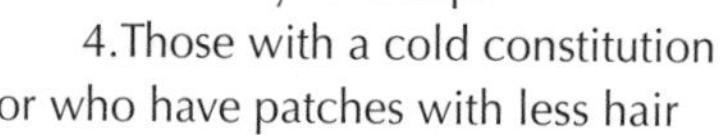

4.Those with a cold constitution or who have patches with less hair growth might use some ginger juice to further stimulate blood flow to the area. Run your fingers through the hair from front to back, with equal pressure over the whole surface of your scalp once again.

contributing to the hair imbalances, for those who are experiencing hair loss in certain patches, or dandruff and itchiness. Apple cider vinegar is one option here. Mix one portion of vinegar to eight portions of warm water. Use the vinegar as a rinse after washing. It can be very helpful against dandruff and helps the hair hold moisture.

- Cooking olives in water then using the tonic water to rinse your hair with can also reduce hair loss and promote hair growth. Make this the final rinse and don't rinse out afterwards (fig. 90).

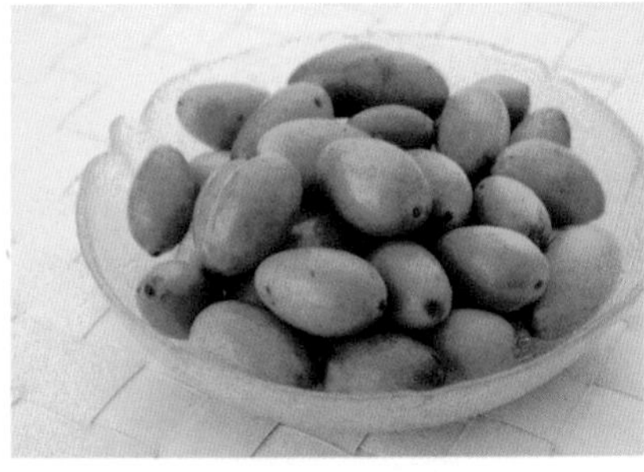

Fig. 90 Olives

- For seborrheic alopecia, you can cook linseed (50 g) and fresh willow branch (50 g) in water and apply the liquid locally, twice a week for two weeks.

Anti-Aging

Aging can wreak havoc on our beauty. Luckily, TCM has many methods for slowing this process.

1) Imbalance: Weaker Teeth

Strong, firm, and white colored teeth make you look more youthful and they frame your smile. Eating too many sweets, not looking after your teeth, and stressful lifestyles can affect the appearance of your teeth.

The kidney controls the storage of essence, your essences stores contribute to your bone marrow, and the bone marrow then dictates the strength and flexibility of your bones. Since the teeth are the outer manifestation of the bones, the strength and health of your teeth are directly influenced by your kidney system. If you have soft teeth that are easily broken or seem to be getting a lot of cavities, despite maintaining good dental hygiene practices, then you may need to strengthen your kidney system.

The following foods are recommended:

- Wolfberry is a fabulous kidney tonic for weak teeth. Adding ten pieces a day to your porridge or hot water (drinking the water and eating the berries) may be helpful. Continue for a 20 day period.

- Making a decoction from the root of drynaria fortune (*gu sui bu*) is another fabulous yang tonic for kidney and teeth. This herb is warm in temperature, bitter in taste, and is a powerful tonic for the kidney and great for strengthening the bones. In fact, it can help to mend bones and stop pain.
- Chinese yam is also a yang tonic for teeth as are macadamia nuts.

2) Imbalance: Hearing Loss or Tinnitus

We have already discussed the relationship between hearing loss and the kidney system.

The following foods are recommended:

- Schisandra berry (Chinese magnolivine fruit, *wu wei zi*) is commonly used to improve hearing function and strengthen the kidney. You may chew the dried berry (six to eight pieces) slowly (for at least three to four minutes) and then swallow them. If you don't like the bitter taste, you could use the berries to make a tea, adding a little honey. It is important to drink both the water and eat the berries. You could take 3 g in a tea and drink two to three cups per day.
- Hearing loss could also be a result of a sinus blockage or ear infection. Turmeric (fig. 91) contains excellent compounds to open the ears. It could also be consumed before a

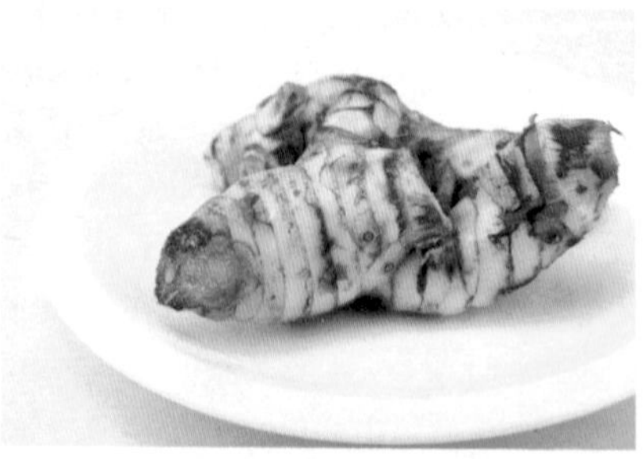

Fig. 91 Fresh turmeric

flight to prevent ear blockages. It can be eaten in food or consumed as a tea.

- Those who are elderly could also make a powder from 150 g of sesame seed and 150 g of mulberry leaf. Mix the powders with brown rice syrup to create pills. Eat 5 g a day for two months.

External remedy:

- You could also rub 20 g of spring onion juice on a tissue and inhale.

3) Imbalance: Joint Weaknesses and Posture

Kidney weakness might cause lower back pain and joint weaknesses, especially in the big joints in the lower body such and the knee and hip (fig. 92).

The following foods are recommended:

- In China, longan fruit is made into a fruit paste or jelly. It is often used as a tonic for these symptoms. You might cook the longan in water until you can mash them into a paste. Alternatively, you could just eat six pieces of dried longan every day throughout the winter.
- Cinnamon is a powerful kidney tonic as is star anise. These spices are eaten more in winter to strengthen yang energy and protect the bones. Cinnamon bark and star anise could be added to cooking, or their powdered form may be sprinkled on top of food. You could

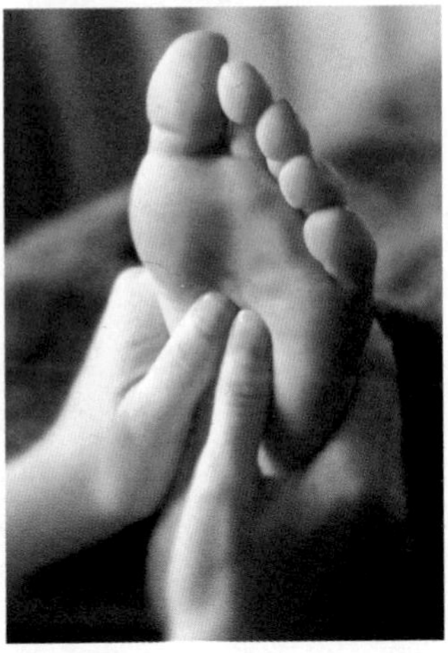

Fig. 92 Pinching your Yongquan point clockwise is helpful for joint weakness.

also use 2 g of cinnamon to add to a tea or if you can find cinnamon tea bags, they may also be used. To strengthen the tonifying effects, 50 g cinnamon bark may be soaked in wine together with 120 g eucommia bark for one month. Then take three times per week in 15 ml dosages during the colder seasons.

- Studies have shown that rice wine or red wine is very good for your joints. Having a shot glass size (10–20 ml) of wine daily with meals can be very tonifying. It is best taken warm, you can heat it up as you would heat up a baby's bottle by placing the dosage in a cup and sitting the cup in hot water until it warms. Rice wine may be substituted for someone who is sensitive to alcohol. Regularly, adding two teaspoons of rice wine while you cook your meals is a good way to include it in the diet.

4) Imbalance: Lower Back Pain

Lower back pain can be caused by poor posture and as we mentioned, posture can be influenced by both the kidney and liver systems of your body. You can decipher whether poor posture is being influenced by the kidney or by the liver based on symptoms.

If the poor posture originates from the kidney, you might find it difficult to stand up straight, even if your mind tells you that it is important to do so. Your bones may be weak and sore, and your spine may ache. Certain conditions where the bones begin to disintegrate may make standing with an impeccable posture very difficult, if not impossible.

If poor posture is originating from the liver, it may be accompanied by an untidy appearance and inability to organize oneself. Along with the gallbladder, your liver helps you make decisions and contributes towards a determined will and mind. Those with a strong liver may decide to stand up tall with a good posture even if it is painful to do so at first, their determination will supersede the pain. Determination of mind is a hallmark of those with a strong liver system. These people will usually be very well dressed and may even dress nicely at home. The liver controls a lot of your natural rhythms, such as menstruation and can contribute to your rhythms of being organized and well presented. Those with a weak liver may not be able to sit or stand up straight, and may go out looking very untidy.

Sex Life

1) Imbalance: Pelvic Floor Dysfunction

Pelvic Floor dysfunction can be a frustrating and embarrassing condition, and it certainly isn't very sexy. In China, there are many natural food remedies and tonics to help with this problem.

The following foods are recommended:

- Euryale seed (fox nut, *qian shi*) is often used to treat pelvic floor dysfunction. It is very good for children, the elderly, and even for men to help prevent them from having spontaneous seminal emission. In China, a Chinese cake is made from the flour that is derived from the crushed seeds. You could also eat it fresh by boiling water, adding the euryale seed, then turning off the heat, and waiting another five minutes before it is ready for consumption. You might sprinkle osmanthus flower to garnish. It can be combined with raspberry to strengthen its properties. Those who are more yin deficient can combine it with lotus seeds.
- Gingko nuts are also effective for stopping vaginal discharge and excessive urination that is caused by weakness in the spleen and kidney. Gingko is an effective functional food, which is commonly used for preventing and treating chronic urine infections, enuresis (bed-wetting), and frequent need to urinate. The dosage is

relative to-age. Children 3-year-old could consume three pieces, 4-year-old may consume four pieces and so on. If continued for seven days, it may be a very effective method for solving bedwetting conditions.

2) Imbalance: Low Sexual Drive

The following foods are recommended:

- Raisins (fig. 93). A few grams of raisins are useful.
- Walnuts have often been used as a tonic for a low sex drive in TCM. You could consume 10 g (three to four pieces) for ten days and this may help to increase sexual desire.
- Clove tea can be made by creating a powder out of fresh cloves and can be taken at night. Place 3–5 g in hot water.
- Pomegranate is warming so those who have a very hot constitution may combine it with some cooling herbs.

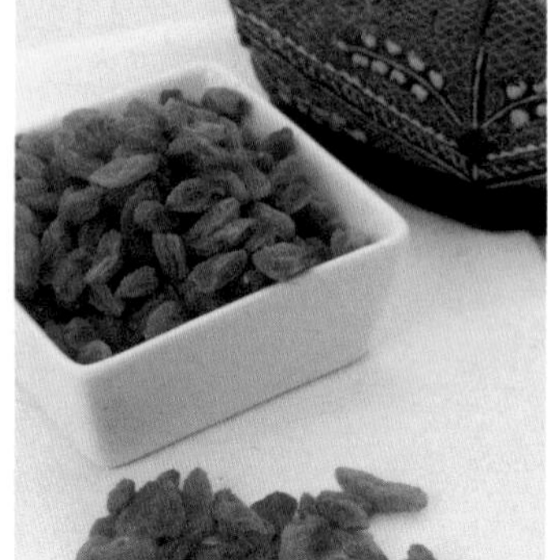

Fig. 93 Raisins

3) Imbalance: Hemorrhoids

Hemorrhoids are another unsexy problem.

The following foods are recommended:

- Kiwi fruit is cool in temperature, and both sweet and sour in nature. It can be helpful for treating hemorrhoids. Thirty to 60 g may be eaten fresh or dried. Dried kiwi can be cooked with rice to make porridge and should be eaten for five days continuously. This can be a useful strategy for pregnant women and can help to reduce the burning pain often experienced in the anal area. This remedy can also

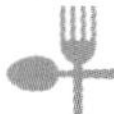

Treat Lung for Hemorrhoids

Figs are effective for reducing and cooling heat. They increase the production of body fluids, aid appetite, dispel swelling, and help to detoxify your system when you have food poisoning. They can treat hemorrhoids, sore throat, hoarseness of voice, and dry cough.

help to quench thirst and combat feelings of overheating.

- A normal serving of wood ear is usually about 5 g. But for hemorrhoids you may need to increase this dosage. Rehydrate 10 g of wood ear, then cook and blend it. Take for five days continuously.

4) Imbalance: Erectile Dysfunction

Men who are finding it hard to get an erection may need to see a doctor to ensure a more serious problem is not present such as prostate disease. The following food remedies can be useful when erectile dysfunction is caused by stress or lifestyle imbalances. In this case, TCM would strengthen the kidney yin and yang.

The following foods are recommended:

- Chive seeds can be powdered and then taken in 6 g dosages in warm water with a little honey or maple syrup.
- Flatstem milkvetch seeds (semen astragali complanati, *sha yuan zi*) can be very useful as they can tonify and warm the liver and kidney, which helps to control seminal emissions.

So your powerful kidney system is responsible for how quickly you age. It supports the proper growth of teeth and bones, and can help you have great posture. Pelvic floor and erectile dysfunctions as well as hemorrhoids. Some types of edema can be remedied by looking after your kidney. Having beautiful hair is another benefit of a well-nourished kidney system. Your kidney works hard to govern and metabolize the fluids in your body. Looking after it will ensure that you remain youthful for life.

APPENDICES

Getting Ready: Preparing Your Kitchen Tools and Ingredients

To get the most out of this book, you should prepare a few things for your kitchen beforehand. The recipes will seem easier if you have a pre-stocked kitchen, making you more likely to start using the recipes to take charge of your health. While there are a few specialty tools and ingredients, for the most part, these are things every cook should have on hand.

Tools

Apart from a basic array of pots and pans, essentials include: a wok, mortar and pestle, steamer with heat-safe ceramic container, and an ovenproof earthenware pot.

Spices

The most important dried spices to keep in your kitchen are: cinnamon (including cinnamon stick), nutmeg, Sichuan pepper, cloves, fennel and dried anise seeds. Dried spices like these can be kept up to two years and therefore only need be replaced when they are used up.

Fresh Ingredients

Remember to pick up fresh spring onion, ginger and garlic whenever you are at the grocery store. Try to purchase ingredients at the local greengrocer, a whole foods or organic store, or at a Chinese grocery. If the fresh ingredients listed in a recipe are not available locally, look for dried, powder or extract forms. These can sometimes even be ordered online. The dosage of these forms should be half that of the fresh.

Sauces and Oils

The following are essential to generating the complex flavors in Chinese cooking and therefore are used for making the soups, stews and other dishes listed in this book: honey, rice wine, oyster sauce, soy sauce, spicy black bean paste, chili sauce, sesame oil, (dark) rice vinegar and apple cider vinegar. Most of them should be covered and kept in a dry, cool and dark place, where they will last for up to a year.

Cooking Techniques

Decoction

Decoction is primarily used for medicinal herbs, such as roots and bark, although it can have more widespread applications.

Wash all the ingredients thoroughly, chop into small pieces if necessary, and put into a cooking pot. Add cold fresh water at a ratio of 8–10:1 (water to dry ingredients). After soaking for a half hour, place pot on the stove and bring to a boil, reducing heat after two minutes to the lowest setting. Herbal decoctions should generally be left on for 30 minutes, although you should follow any specific directions given in a recipe. Fifteen minutes are needed for a small quantity of leaves or flowers or for a recipe for acute flu or cold. For a meat decoction, check the doneness of the meat; one hour is usually required.

When finished, strain the decoction, preserving the liquid. If seeds or other materials pass through the strainer, use a fine strainer, again preserving the liquid. Most herbal decoctions need to be boiled again, reducing heat to low after two minutes. In this second round, it should be allowed to simmer for 10 to 20 minutes. Split into multiple portions if necessary, and drink warm.

Fruit Wine

To make a fruit wine, buy Chinese distilled liquor (50%) and the prescribed fruit. Separate the rice wine into two bottles, and add half of the fruit to each bottle. The ratio of wine to fruit should be 2:1. Store for ten days to one month in the dark, after which it will be ready to drink.

Soup

Prepare all the ingredients, washing, soaking and chopping into bite-sized pieces as needed. Put fresh water and ingredients into a large cooking pot (enamel preferred), and bring to a boil. For a meat soup, add ginger and rice wine once boiling. Reduce to a simmer for 20 minutes to an hour depending on ingredients (vegetables will take less time than meat). Add spring onion and any other flavoring ten minutes before done.

Steaming

In a large pot, add enough water that it won't entirely boil away but not so much that it touches the steaming basket (usually two inches will work). Bring to a boil, then place the steaming basket with ingredients spread evenly over the boiling water. Place the lid on the large pot, and don't open, unless necessary.

For vegetables, steam until tender, about 8–15 minutes. For 250 g of fish, steam for ten minutes; with each additional 250 g of fish, add five minutes of steaming time. For meat, steam for about 20–30 minutes until cooked thoroughly. When the time is up, turn off the burner, but leave the lid on for another few minutes.

A recipe may call for using a heat-safe ceramic or glass container to steam. Take note whether the ceramic container should have a perforated lid or no lid. Then place the lid on the large pot and allow to steam. The typical quantity for ceramic steaming is 25–50 g. Steaming ginseng or other roots requires at least 45 minutes to one hour.

Paste

When making paste, the total weight of the ingredients should be at least 500–750 g, with each item being at least 50 g. To make a paste, you will follow the same basic procedure as for a decoction: wash, boil, strain, repeat.

For the first round, the ratio of water to ingredients is 6:1. After the first boiling, strain the liquid and keep it separated. Then add water to the original ingredients, at a 5:1 ratio this time, and boil again. Strain, and add the new liquid to the previous liquid. Then, using a 4:1 ratio, boil, strain and add this to existing liquid, discarding all the solids. Use a cloth strainer and strain the combined liquid once more.

Place the strained liquid in a cooking pot and use medium-low heat to reduce further. Once the water has mostly boiled off and it has become sticky, add honey to taste. Remove from heat and store in a glass or ceramic container in the refrigerator. For most pastes, you will eat one tablespoon a day, spreading it on toast or adding to hot water for a syrupy drink.

Porridge

Put water and ingredients in a pot, with a 6:1 ratio of water to ingredients. Bring to a boil, then after two minutes, reduce to a simmer. Cover with a lid (with some ventilation, most rice cookers come with a small hole or vent); stir only once. For oats, simmer for 20 minutes. For brown rice, simmer for 40 minutes.

Meridian Database: Illustrations, Acupuncture Points and Locations

According to traditional Chinese medicine, acupuncture points are tiny spots where qi and blood are infused in meridians, collaterals and internal organs. They are not only reaction points of diseases, but also stimulation points for acupuncture, moxibustion and other treatment.

Inside the human body, there are 12 "regular" meridians in total. Adding in the Conception Vessel at the front center of the body and the Governing Vessel at the rear center, we will discuss 14 meridians in this book. A total of 365 acupuncture points are arranged along them.

Please note that each meridian circulates along two lines: the inside line and the outside line. The connections between meridian's inside lines and the organs are quite exquisite and diversified. Since this book is mainly for beauty, we only discuss the more related outside lines.

There are many acupuncture points not included in the fourteen meridians that have important efficacies as well as explicit locations and names. These are called "irregular" acupuncture points. This book also introduces some irregular acupuncture points often used as a means of prevention and treatment.

In naming meridians/collaterals and acupuncture points, this books uses codes from the standard of World Federation of Chinese Medicine Societies—Specialty Committee of Publishers and Editors, namely: abbreviations of meridian/collateral names

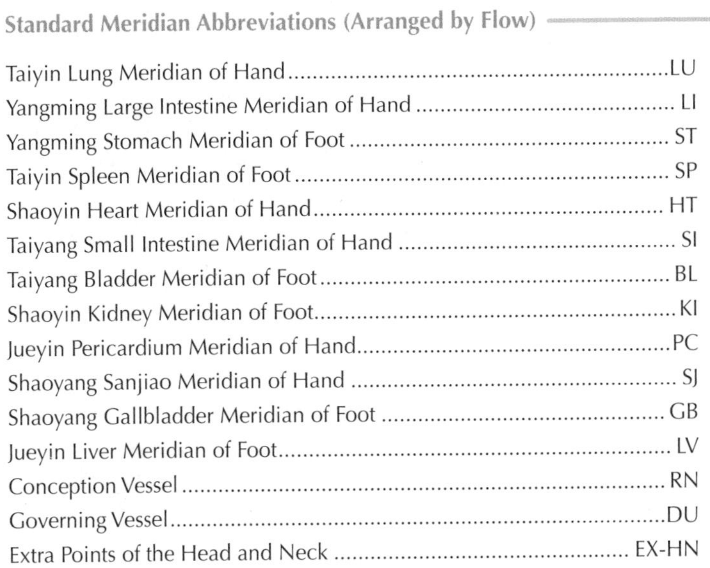

Standard Meridian Abbreviations (Arranged by Flow)

Taiyin Lung Meridian of Hand .... LU
Yangming Large Intestine Meridian of Hand LI
Yangming Stomach Meridian of Foot .... ST
Taiyin Spleen Meridian of Foot .... SP
Shaoyin Heart Meridian of Hand .... HT
Taiyang Small Intestine Meridian of Hand .... SI
Taiyang Bladder Meridian of Foot .... BL
Shaoyin Kidney Meridian of Foot .... KI
Jueyin Pericardium Meridian of Hand .... PC
Shaoyang Sanjiao Meridian of Hand .... SJ
Shaoyang Gallbladder Meridian of Foot .... GB
Jueyin Liver Meridian of Foot LV
Conception Vessel .... RN
Governing Vessel .... DU
Extra Points of the Head and Neck .... EX-HN

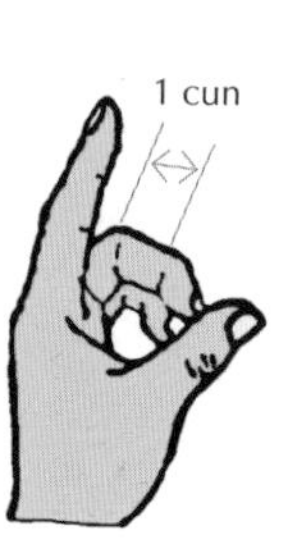

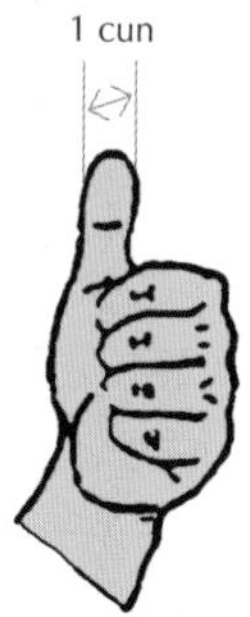

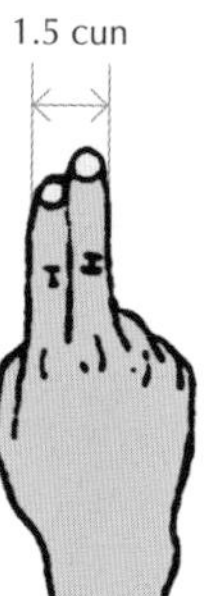

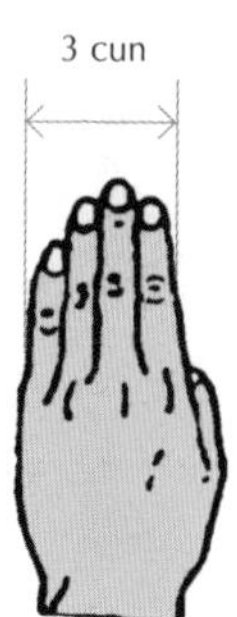

plus serial numbers.

For acupuncture point names, Chinese pinyin names (transliterated names) and Chinese characters are used. The names often have deep links to Chinese classical culture and profound meanings.

This table also lists the locations of acupuncture points so that readers can find them conveniently. An important means of location is the "cun" measurements of the body. This system is an ingenious way by which anyone can measure and locate acupoints on his or her own body. Since everyone's body is of a different size and shape, using a measurement system specific to the individual makes finding the points easy.

The process starts with the measurement of one cun. This is done in two ways:

- Using the width of the distal inter-phalangeal joint of the thumb
- Using the distance between the distal and proximal inter-phalangeal joints of the third (middle) finger.

All other specific measurements are outlined in the diagrams below. When in doubt in measuring, the thumb (1 cun) or the four finger method (3 cun) can always be used.

1. Shaoyin Heart Meridian of Hand (HT) (Heart System)

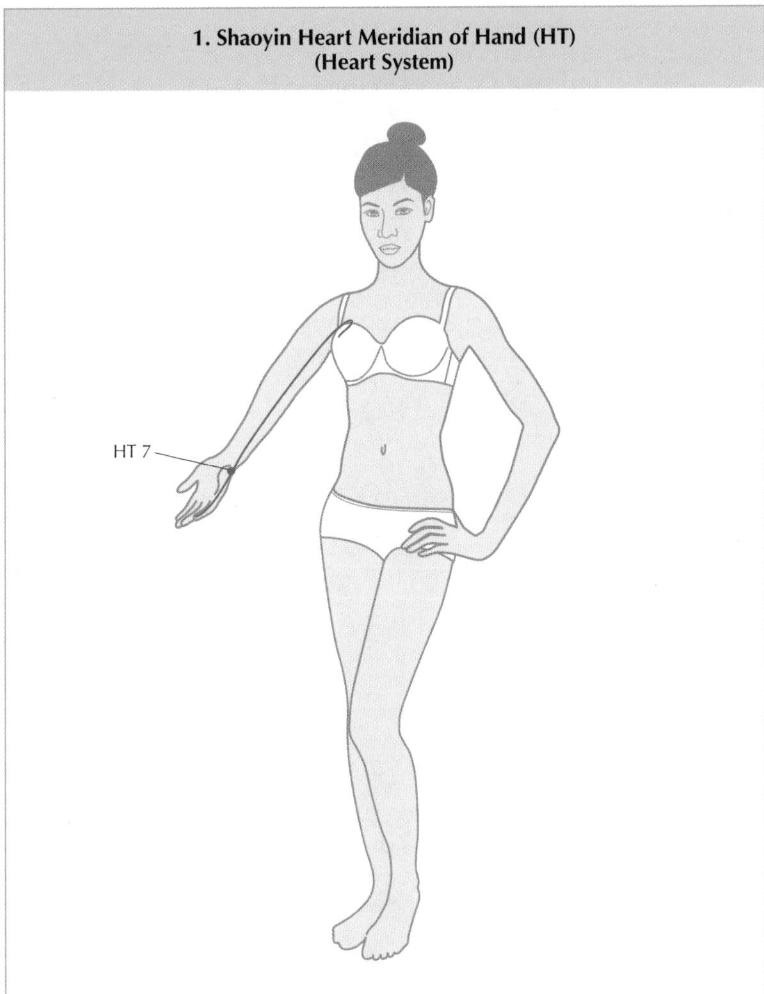

<table>
<tr><th rowspan="2">Code</th><th colspan="2">Name of Acupoint</th><th rowspan="2">Location</th></tr>
<tr><th>Pinyin and Chinese</th><th>Translation</th></tr>
<tr><td>HT 7</td><td>Shenmen point
神门穴</td><td>Spirit Gate</td><td>On the ulnar side of the transverse wrist crease, in the depression on the radial ulnar wrist flexor tendon</td></tr>
</table>

2. Taiyang Small Intestine Meridian of Hand (SI)
(Heart System)

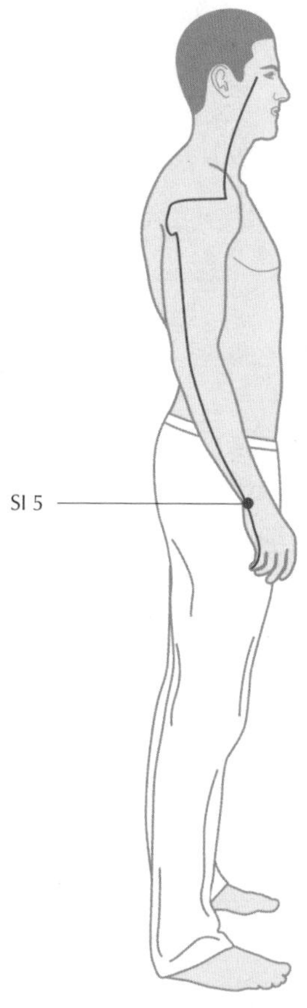

Code	Name of Acupoint		Location
	Pinyin and Chinese	Translation	
SI 5	Yanggu point 阳谷穴	Yang Valley	On the ulnar aspect of the wrist, in the depression between the styloid process of the ulna and the triquetral bone.

3. Jueyin Pericardium Meridian of Hand (PC) (Heart System)

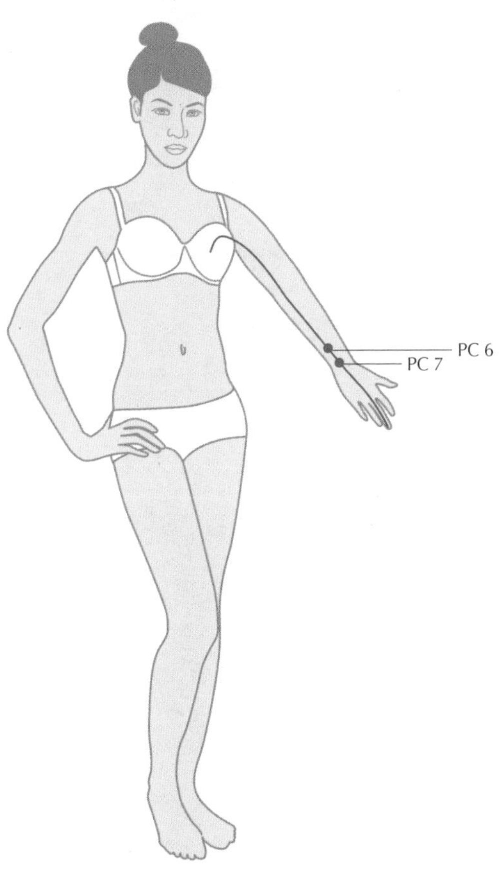

Code	Name of Acupoint		Location
	Pinyin and Chinese	Translation	
PC 6	Neiguan point 内关穴	Inner Gate	Between two tendons, 2 cun over the wrist transverse crease
PC 7	Daling point 大陵穴	Big Mound	Between two tendons at the midpoint of the wrist and palm transverse crease

4. Shaoyang *San Jiao* Meridian of Hand (SJ) (Heart System)

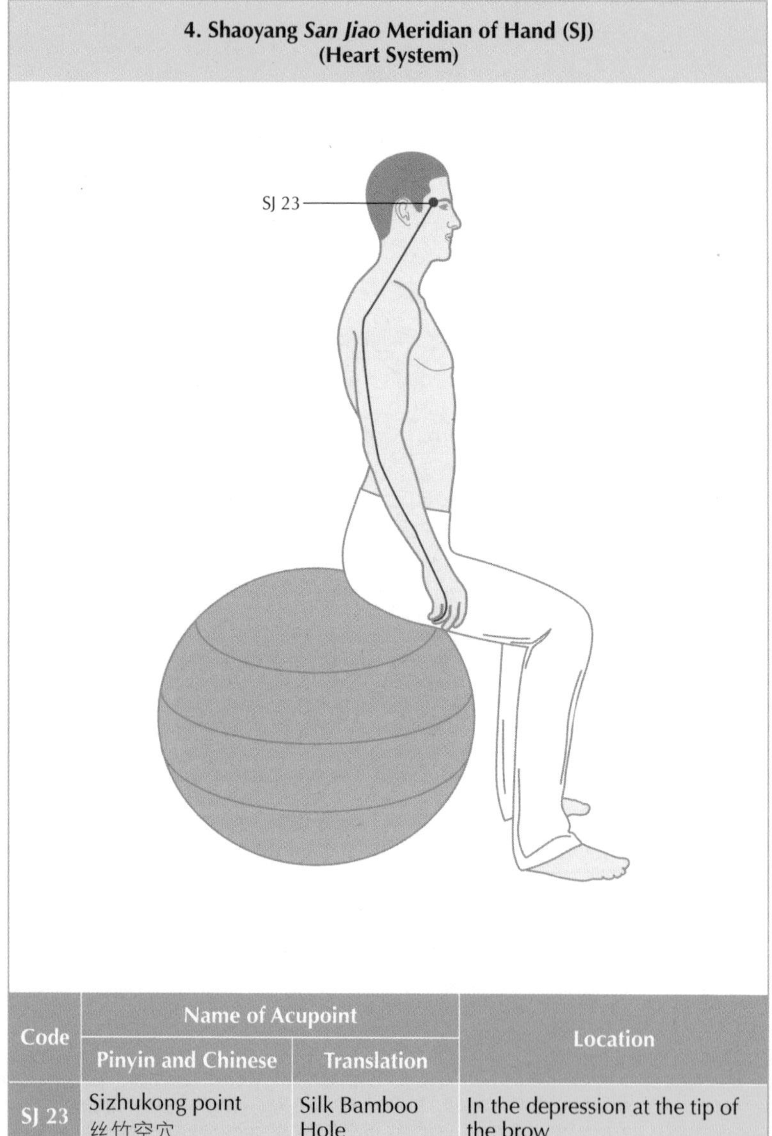

Code	Name of Acupoint		Location
	Pinyin and Chinese	Translation	
SJ 23	Sizhukong point 丝竹空穴	Silk Bamboo Hole	In the depression at the tip of the brow

5. Taiyin Lung Meridian of Hand (LU)
(Lung System)

LU1

Code	Name of Acupoint		Location
	Pinyin and Chinese	Translation	
LU 1	Zhongfu point 中府穴	Middle Storehouse	6 cun horizontally away from the front central line; in the superior lateral part of the anterior thoracic wall, in the intercostal space of the first rib

6. Yangming Large Intestine Meridian of Hand (LI)
(Lung System)

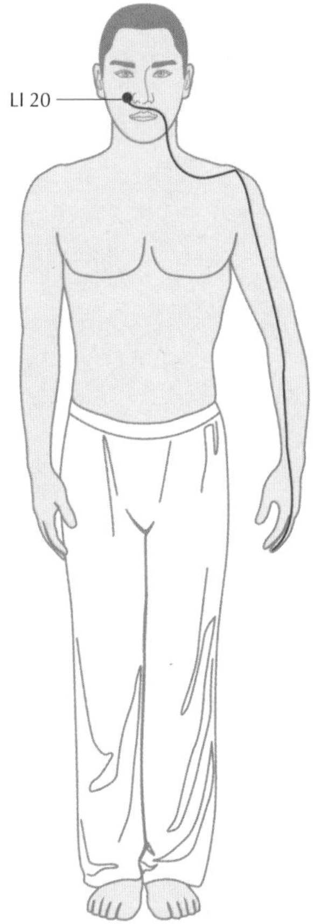

LI 20

Code	Name of Acupoint		Location
	Pinyin and Chinese	Translation	
LI 20	Yingxiang point 迎香穴	Welcoming Perfume	0.5 cun beside the wing of nose, in the nasolabial groove

7. Jueyin Liver Meridian of Foot (LV)
(Liver System)

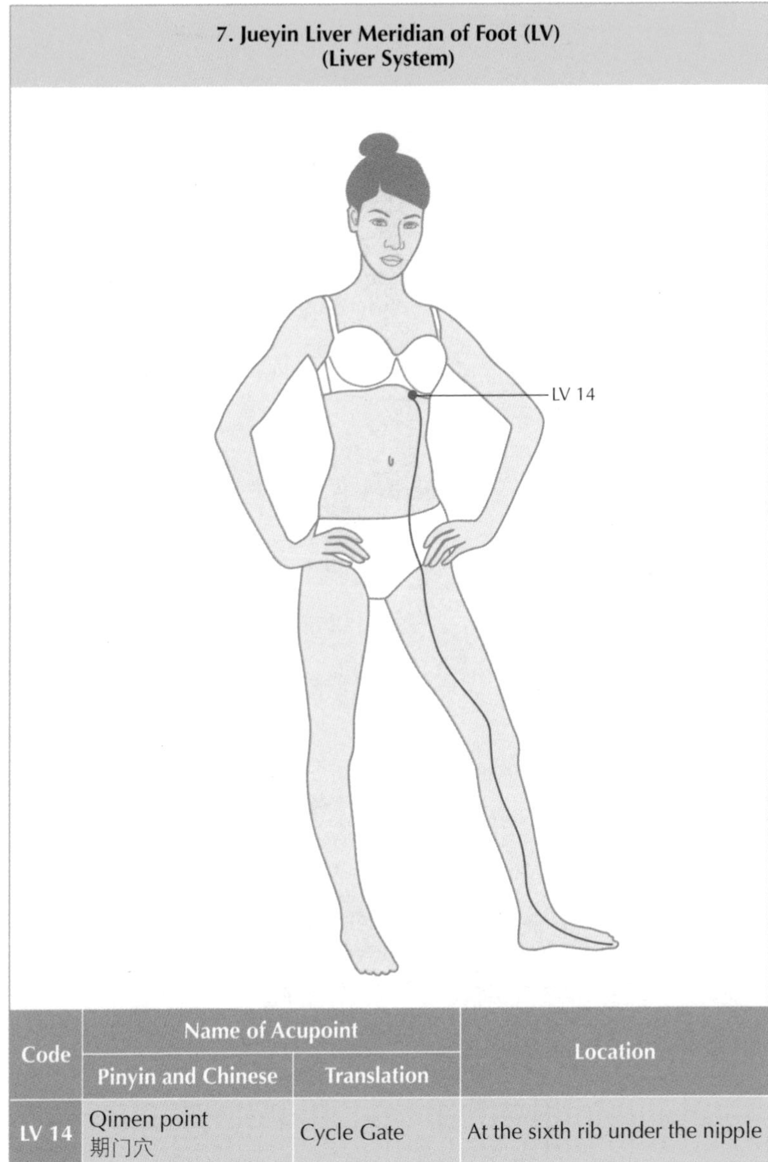

Code	Name of Acupoint		Location
	Pinyin and Chinese	Translation	
LV 14	Qimen point 期门穴	Cycle Gate	At the sixth rib under the nipple

8. Shaoyang Gallbladder Meridian of Foot (GB)
(Liver System)

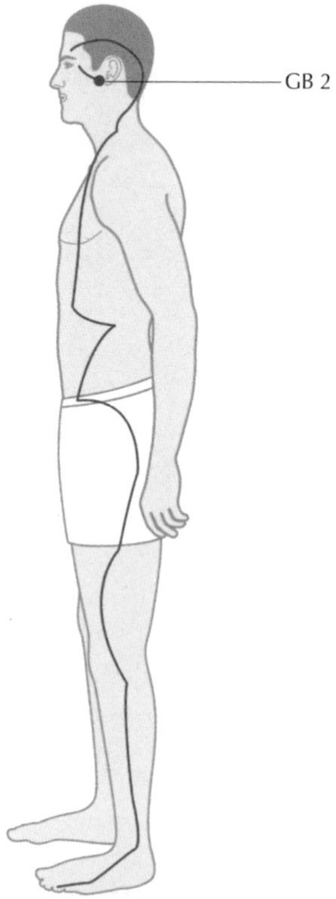

GB 2

Code	Name of Acupoint		Location
	Pinyin and Chinese	Translation	
GB 2	Tinghui point 听会穴	Reunion of Hearing	In front of the indentation of the antilobium

9. Taiyin Spleen Meridian of Foot (SP) (Spleen System)

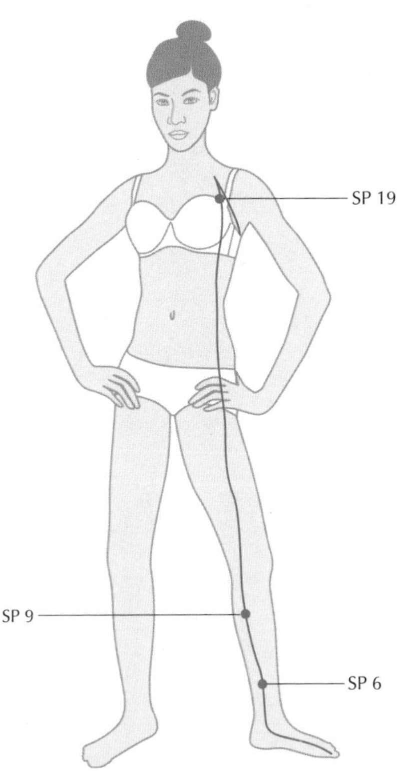

Code	Name of Acupoint		Location
	Pinyin and Chinese	Translation	
SP 6	Sanyinjiao point 三阴交穴	Three Yin Intersection	On the rear edge of the shin bone, 3 cun above the ankle
SP 9	Yinlingquan point 阴陵泉穴	Shady Side of the Mountain	In the depression on the inner edge of the shin bone by the knee
SP 19	Xiongxiang point 胸乡穴	Chest Village	On the lateral aspect of the chest, in the 3rd intercostal space, 6 cun from the anterior midline of the body

10. Yangming Stomach Meridian of Foot (ST)
(Spleen System)

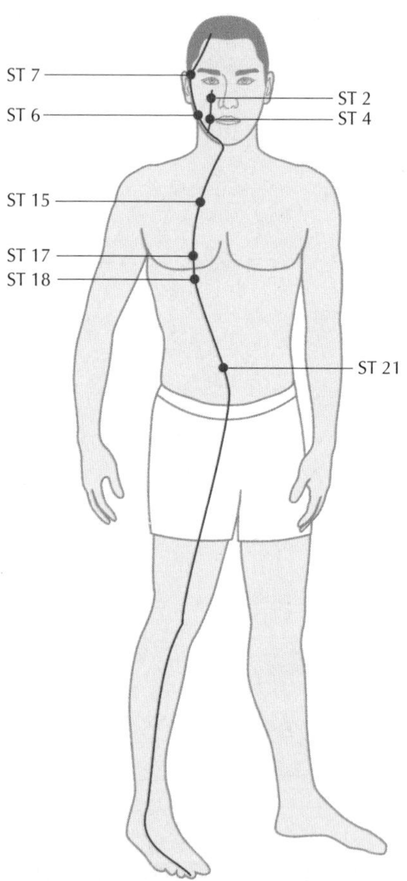

Code	Name of Acupoint		Location
	Pinyin and Chinese	Translation	
ST 2	Sibai point 四白穴	Four Whites	In the depression of the orifice under the eye socket, under the central line of the eyeball

Code	Name of Acupoint		Location
	Pinyin and Chinese	Translation	
ST 6	Jiache point 颊车穴	Jaw Chariot (Jawbone)	In the depression one horizontal finger from the upper front of the angle of the mandible; this will crease when the teeth are clenched
ST 7	Xiaguan point 下关穴	Below the Joint	In the depression at the hair line in front of the ear; it can be felt when the mouth is closed and creases when the mouth is open
ST 15	Wuyi point 屋翳穴	Stomach Roof	On the chest, in the 2nd intercostal space, 4 cun lateral to the anterior median line.
ST 17	Ruzhong point 乳中穴	Breast Center	At the center of the nipple
ST 18	Rugen point 乳根穴	Breast Root	At the base of the breast under the nipple
ST 21	Liangmen point 梁门穴	Beam Gate	On the upper abdomen, four cun above the center of the umbilicus and 2 cun lateral to the anterior midline.

11. Shaoyin Kidney Meridian of Foot (KI)
(Kidney System)

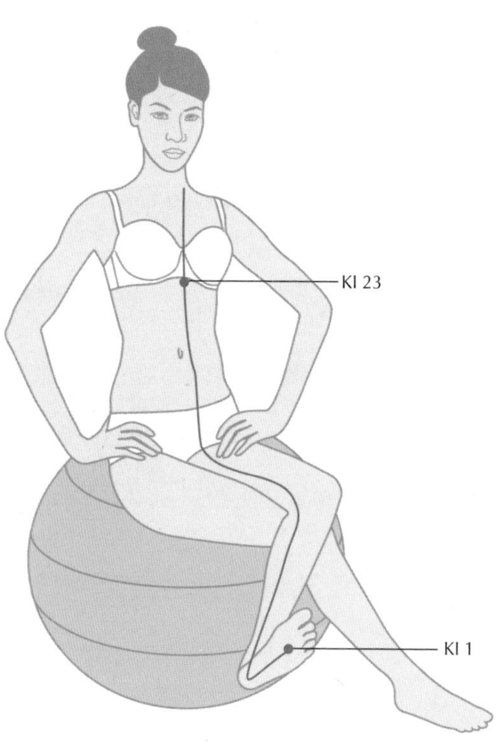

<table>
<tr><th rowspan="2">Code</th><th colspan="2">Name of Acupoint</th><th rowspan="2">Location</th></tr>
<tr><th>Pinyin and Chinese</th><th>Translation</th></tr>
<tr><td>KI 1</td><td>Yongquan point
涌泉穴</td><td>Bubbling Spring</td><td>In the depression in the front of the sole</td></tr>
<tr><td>KI 23</td><td>Shenfeng point
神封穴</td><td>Spirit Seal</td><td>On the chest, in the 4th intercostal space, 2 cun lateral to the anterior midline</td></tr>
</table>

12. Taiyang Bladder Meridian of Foot (BL)
(Kidney System)

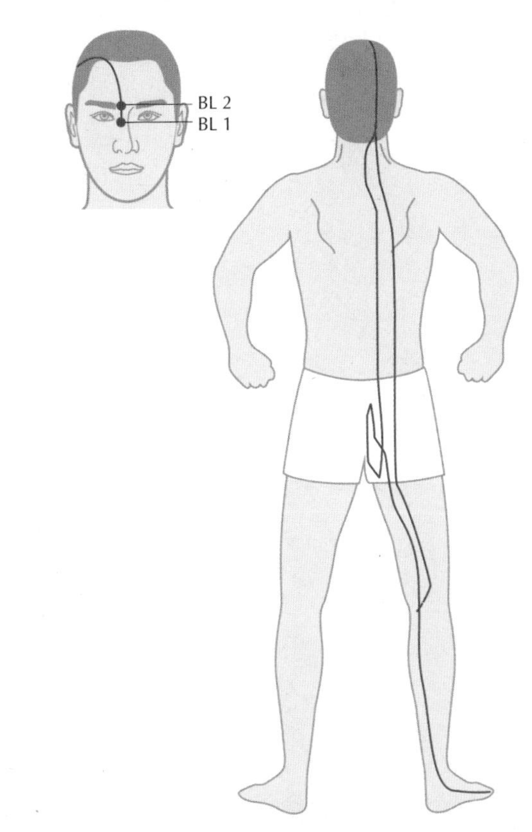

Code	Name of Acupoint		Location
	Pinyin and Chinese	Translation	
BL 1	Jingming point 睛明穴	Bright Eyes	In the depression 0.1 cun over the inner corner of eye
BL 2	Cuanzhu point 攒竹穴	Bamboo Gathering	On the edge of the eye socket, on the inner edge of the eyebrow

13. Conception Vessel (RN)

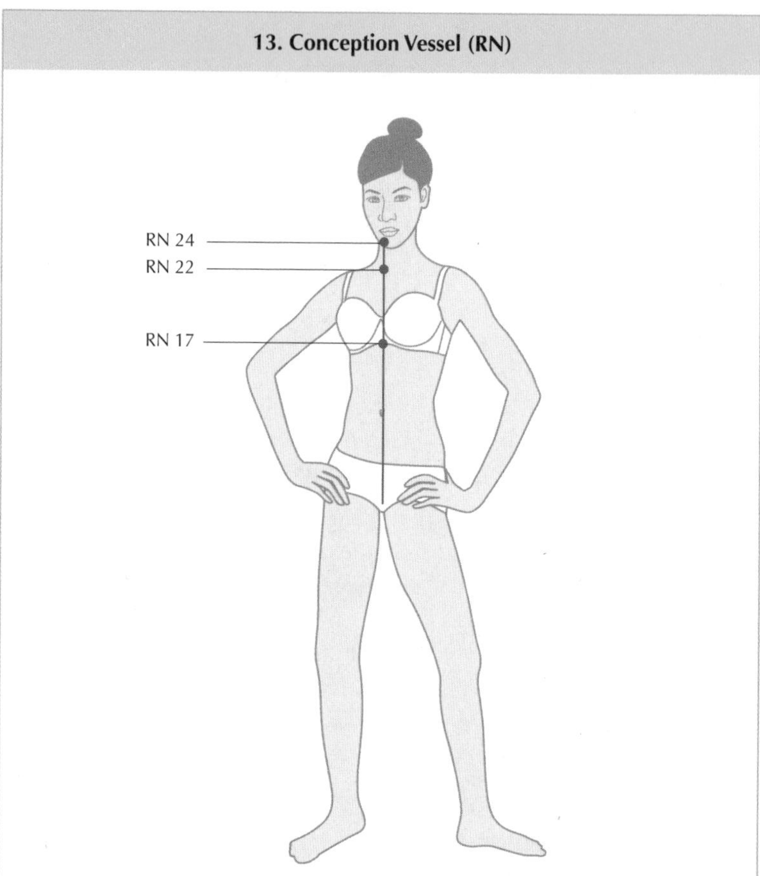

Code	Name of Acupoint		Location
	Pinyin and Chinese	Translation	
RN 17	Danzhong point 膻中穴	Sea of Tranquility	Parallel with the intercostal space of the fourth rib; at the front central line
RN 22	Tiantu point 天突穴	Heaven Rushing Out, Sun Point	At the center of the suprasternal fossa
RN 24	Chengjiang point 承浆穴	Sauce Receptacle	In the depression at the center of the mentolabial sulcus of the face

14. Governing Vessel (DU)

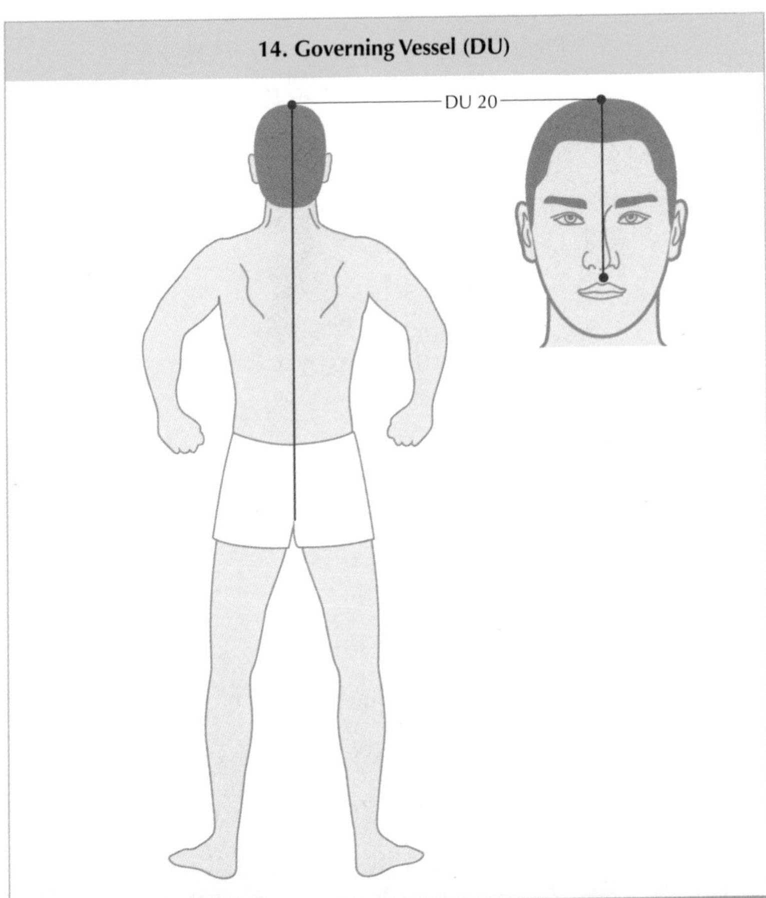

Code	Name of Acupoint		Location
	Pinyin and Chinese	Translation	
DU 20	Baihui point 百会穴	One Hundred Meeting Point	At the center of the skull, over the two ear tips
DU 26	Shuigou point 水沟穴	Water Trough	In the recessed grove at the center between the nose and upper lip

15. Extra Points of the Head and Neck (EX-HN)

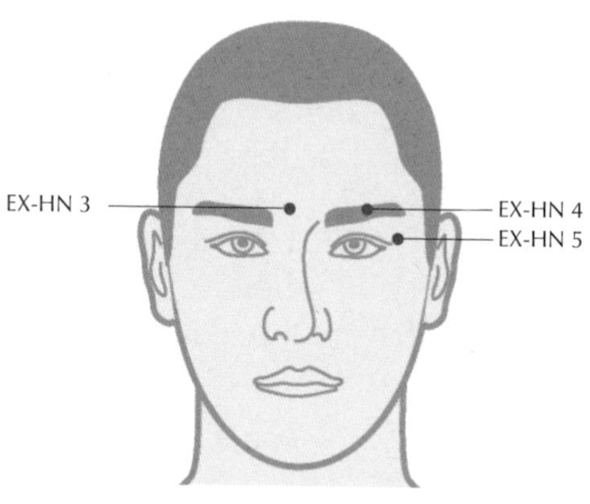

Code	Name of Acupoint		Location
	Pinyin and Chinese	Translation	
EX-HN 3	Yintang point 印堂穴	Hall of Seal	At the midpoint of the line connecting the two brows
EX-HN 4	Yuyao point 鱼腰穴	Fish Loin	In the middle of the eyebrow.
EX-HN 5	Taiyang point 太阳穴	Temple	In the depression about 1 cun behind the space between the outer tip of the brow and outer eye corner

TCM Glossary

Body Constitution 体质

Body constitution is formed before birth but can be influenced by factors after birth. The constitution comprises features of the body's structure and its physiological and psychological functions.

Body Fluid 津液

Body fluid in TCM is a general term for all normal liquids in the body. It is one of the essential substances of the human body and vital to maintaining life activities. Body fluid and blood are both derived from the essence of the foods you consume. Body fluid is a component of blood, and the two substances can transform into each other. Thus it is said: "body fluid and blood share the same source."

Chinese Herbal Medicine 中草药

In China, herbs are the primary therapeutic agent of internal medicine. Of the approximately 1000 herbs utilized today, 500 or so are very commonly used. Rather than being prescribed individually, herbs are usually combined into formulas, containing 2–25 herbs, which are adapted to the specific needs of the patient. As with functional foods, each herb has one or more of the five "tastes" (sweet, sour, salty, spicy, bitter) and one of the five "energies" or temperatures (hot, warm, neutral, cool, cold). After the herbalist determines the properties of the patient's body, he or she prescribes a mixture of herbs tailored to balance disharmony.

Congenital Base of Life 肾为先天之本

The body's constitution as determined before birth is controlled by the kidney and its function.

Congenital Natural Disposition 先天禀赋

In addition to the kidney, prenatal influences on the constitution include the state of nutrition and other influences on development. The health of the mother during pregnancy has an effect on the constitution.

Dietary (Food) Therapy 食疗

Dietary recommendations are usually made according to the patient's individual condition in relation to TCM theory. This relates to the "four energies" (hot, warm, cold and cool plus neutral) and "five tastes", which are also important aspects of Chinese herbal medicine. These determine what effects various types of food have on the body. A balanced diet leading to health is achieved when the energies and tastes are in balance. When one gets disease (and is therefore unbalanced), certain formerly routine foods must be avoided or reduced while some new ones must be added to restore balance in the body.

Essence 精

Essence, one of the most valuable components of the human body, consists of two aspects. The first refers to the basic material that forms the viscera, tissues, skin, hair, tendons and muscles. The second refers to the reproductive essence, which comprises not only the individual's own reproductive essence but also the hereditary reproductive essence (ie that of the parents). The kidney has the function of preserving and storing essence.

Five Emotions 五志

The five emotions are matched with the five *zang*-organs: the heart governs joy, the liver governs anger, the lung governs worry, the spleen governs thinking, and the kidney governs fear.

Kidney-Yin and Kidney-Yang 肾阴肾阳

These are also called the primordial or true yin (true water) and primordial or true yang (true fire). Kidney-yin is the foundation of the yin-fluid of the entire body, moistening and nourishing the tissues and organs. Kidney-yang is the foundation of the body's yang-qi, which has warming functions and promotes the growth of tissues and organs. Therefore kidney-yin and kidney-yang are the source of yin and yang in all other organs.

Meridians and Collaterals 经络

Meridians and collaterals are pathways through which qi and blood circulate and through which the viscera and limbs are connected. They allow communication between the upper and lower parts of the body as well as the interior and exterior.

Property Transformation (Transformation According to Constitution) 从化

This principle states that the same environment will lead to different outcomes and diseases based on differences in body constitution.

Qi 气

Qi is the most fundamental substance of the human body. It is the energy or life-process that flows in and around all of us. There are four kinds of qi:

Original qi (*yuan qi*, 元气): Original qi is closely related to essence from congenital. It also enriches and relies on acquired essence. It passes through the *san jiao* and spreads to the internal organs and meridians. It's one of the most important qi.

Chest qi (*zong qi*, 宗气): Qi that accumulates in the chest. It nourishes and supports the heart and lung. It is composed of clear air inhaled by the lung and the essence that is transformed by the stomach and spleen from food.

Nutrition qi (*ying qi*, 营气): This nourishing qi flows in the inner layers and the internal organs (e.g. blood vessels with in the channels). It comes mainly from the nutritive part (yin temperature and taste) of the food.

Defensive qi (*wei qi*, 卫气): The qi flows on the outer layers of the body (outside of the vessels with in the channels). It has a protective function. It is more yang compared with nutrition qi. It comes mainly from the vigorous part of the food (yang temperature and taste).

Qi Activity, Qi Transformation 气机、气化

The movement of qi is called "qi activity". The various changes associated with movements of qi are called "qi transformation".

Source of Acquired Constitution 后天之本

While the kidney is the congenital foundation of constitution, the spleen is the source of acquired constitution. The spleen system directs food transport and transformation, playing a role in digestion and assimilation of nutrients. These functions play an important role in the formation of qi and blood.

Spirit 神

In TCM theory, the term "spirit" is an abstract concept. In the broad sense, it encompasses the outward activities of life, and refers to the comprehensive whole. This includes the vitality of the body, appearance, complexion, expression of the eyes, speech, responsiveness, etc. In the narrow sense, spirit is a collective term for cognition, consciousness and other mental activities.

San Jiao 三焦

San jiao is the collective term for the three sections of the body, known as the upper, middle, and lower *jiao*. It is one of the six *fu* organs.

TCM Body Clock 十二时辰

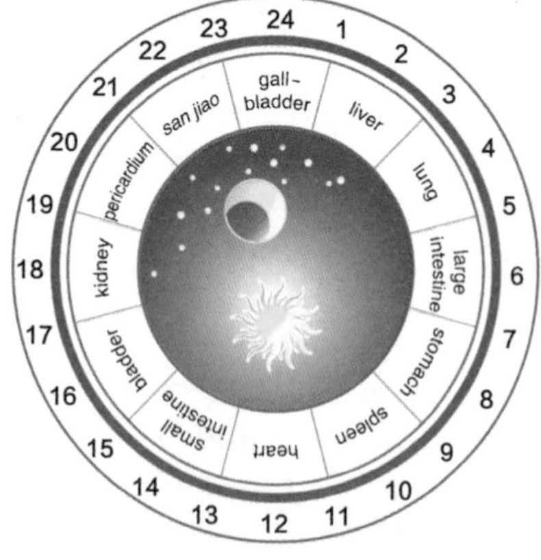

The day is broken down into two-hour periods, each related to specific organs, meridians, functions and recommended behaviors.

Chou (1–3 a.m.): The liver meridian is on duty to dispel toxins and produce fresh new blood in liver.

Yin (3–5 a.m.): The lung meridian distributes the energy and blood produced by the liver to the organs.

Mao (5–7 a.m.): During these two hours, one should sit next to a window in the light, drink a cup of warm water (rather than tea) and comb the hair and head repeatedly. This helps dispel pathogenic energies in the body and clear the eyesight and the mind. It is also the time to wash.

Chen (7–9 a.m.): This is the time for breakfast since the stomach meridian is active. With sufficient yang energy from food, the spleen then turns nutrients into energy and leaves no extra fat to accumulate (if one doesn't overeat).

Si (9–11 a.m.): Blood and energy flow to the spleen meridian supporting metabolism. Nutrients are converted into blood and energy, and sent to the muscles. This is a prime time for working since the energy and blood distributed by the spleen will support activity.

Wu (11–1 p.m.): A balanced, nutritious lunch is important; it shouldn't be too big. Take a slow walk after lunch and rub the stomach and lower back to get the spleen and kidney active. Drinking a little tea and taking a half hour's nap is recommended.

Wei (1–3 p.m.): After lunch and a nap (no more than an hour), it is time for more activity, as the small intestine works to separate and distribute digested nutrients.

Shen (3–5 p.m.): The two bladder meridians go to work, one on each side of the spine, running from the foot to the head. Since energy and blood flow into the brain, it is a good time for efficient work and study. Afternoon tea is recommended. The bladder meridian is also a major toxin-expelling channel and handles toxins dispelled by other meridians. Drinking extra water allows toxins to be passed in urine.

You (5–7 p.m.): The kidney starts to store "essence" as the kidney meridian takes its turn. This is the best time for kidney-reinforcing therapy. It's time for dinner but not too much. A little wine is good to activate blood circulation.

Xu (7–9 p.m.): The pericardium is the fluid-filled sac that surrounds the heart and the roots of major blood vessels. It contains channels of blood and energy. When it is activated at xu, it dispels all the pathogenic energy around the heart to protect it. At this time it's advised to soak the feet in hot water, which can help dispel pathogenic heat and damp, activating blood circulation. Massaging the yong quan point (the arch of foot) in both feet can help nourish kidney energy.

Hai (9–11 p.m.) and Zi (11 p.m.–1 a.m.): Zi is the darkest hour when strong yin energy starts to fade and yang energy begins to grow. Sufficient yang energy allows people to stay active during the day, so it should be well-stored at the right time. Since sleep is the best way to store yang energy, it is best to be in deep sleep at zi, which means you should go to sleep at hai. People should not go outdoors from hai to zi. Hai is also the best time of the day for sex (also for getting pregnant), when yin and yang are in balance in the body and in the universe.

Yin-Yang 阴阳

Yin and yang are the two fundamental principles or forces in the universe, opposing and supplementing each other. Yin includes blood, body fluid and visible material; yang includes qi, the functions of the body, and invisible material.

Zang-Fu Organs 脏腑

The internal organs of the human body are called the *zang-fu* organs.

Five *zang*-organs (五脏): The heart, lung, spleen, liver and kidney are known as the five *zang*-organs.

Six *fu*-organs (六腑): The gallbladder, stomach, small intestine, large intestine, urinary bladder and *san jiao* are called the six-*fu* organs.

Five *zang-fu* systems (五脏系统): These systems each have one of the five *zang*-organs as the center, from which stem internal links with the *fu*-organs. They are further externally connected with the limbs and tissues, the five sense organs and their manifestations.

Extraordinary *fu*-organs (奇恒之腑): Called "qi hen" denoting extraordinary, these are the brain, marrow, bone, blood vessels, gallbladder and uterus.

Relationship between *zang-fu* organs (脏腑表里关系): "*Zang*" pertains to yin while "*fu*" pertains to yang. Therefore, the relationships between the *zang*-organs and the *fu*-organs refer to yin-yang and exterior-interior relationships.

Bibliography

English:

1. Zhang Yifang. *Managing Your Emotional Health Using Traditional Chinese Medicine*. New York: Reader's Digest, 2010.
2. Zhang Yifang & Yao Yingzhi. *Your Guide to Health with Foods & Herbs: Using the Wisdom of Traditional Chinese Medicine*. New York: Better Link Press, 2012.
3. Zhang Enqin, Shi Lanhua etc. *Basic Theory of Traditional Chinese Medicine*. Shanghai: Publishing House of Shanghai College of Traditional Chinese Medicine, 1990.
4. Zuo Yanfu, Tang Decai. *Science of Chinese Materia Medica*. Shanghai: Publishing House of Shanghai University of Traditional Chinese Medicine, 2003.
5. Cheng Xinnong. *Chinese Acupuncture and Moxibustion*. Beijing: Foreign Languages Press, 1987.
6. Wiseman etc. *Fundamentals of Chinese Medicine, Revised edition*. US: Paradigm Publications, 1996.
7. Zhang Enqin, Zhang Wengao etc. *Chinese Medicated Diet*. Shanghai: Publishing House of Shanghai College of Traditional Chinese Medicine, 1990.
8. Zuo Yanfu, Wu Changguo. *Basic Theory of Traditional Chinese Medicine*. Shanghai: Publishing House of Shanghai University of Traditional Chinese Medicine, 2003.
9. Beijing University of Traditional Chinese Medicine. *Basic Theories of Traditional Chinese Medicine*. Beijing: Academy Press, 1998.
10. Zhang Qian. *The TCM Body Clock*. Shanghai: *Shanghai Daily*, 21 December, 2010, p. B1-2.
11. Deborah Mitchell. *The Complete Book of Nutritional Healing*. US: St. Martin's Paperbacks edition, 2009.
12. Library of Chinese Classics. *Yellow Emperor's Canon of Medicine, Plain Conversation*. Xi'an: World Publishing Corporation, 2005.

13. Giovanni Maciocia. *The Foundations of Chinese Medicine*. London: Churchill Livingstone, 1989.
14. Daverick Leggett. *Helping Ourselves a Guide to Traditional Chinese Food Energetics*. England: Meridian Press, 1994.
15. Nicola Peterson, *Herbs and Health*. London: Bloomsbury books, 1993.

中文：

1. 张继泽等:《张泽生医案医话集》,江苏科技出版社,1981年。
2. 张挹芳:《中医藏象学》,中国协和医科大学出版社,2004年。
3. 张挹芳:《孟河传人张泽生张继泽中医承启集》,东南大学出版社,2010年。
4. 张杰:《胃肠病药膳良方》,人民卫生出版社,2002年。
5. 唐传核:《植物功能性食品》,化学工业出版社,2004年。
6. 陈士林等:《中草药大典》,军事医学科学出版社,2006年
7. 彭铭泉:《大众药膳煲》,四川科学技术出版社,1995年。
8. 罗丹妮:《本草纲目中的美容养颜经》,朝华出版社,2009年。
9. 傅杰英:《美啊,请你停一停——中医体质美容使用手册》,江苏人民出版社,2010年。
10. 匡调元:《人体体质学——理论应用和发展》,上海中医学院出版社,1991年。
11. 窦国祥:《饮食治疗指南》,江苏科学技术出版社,1981年。
12. 南京中医学院中医系:《黄帝内经灵枢译释》,上海科学技术出版社,1986年。
13. 南京中医药大学:《中药大辞典》,上海科学技术出版社,2006年。

Index

A

absent-mindedness 84
acupressure/acupuncture point
  Baihui point (DU 20) 230–231, 270, 299
  Chengjiang point (RN 24) 155, 231, 298
  Cuanzhu point (BL 2) 155, 230–231, 297
  Daling point (PC 7) 134, 287
  Danzhong point (RN 17) 163, 217, 298
  Dicang point (ST 4) 231
  Jiache point (ST 6) 231, 295
  Jingming point (BL 1) 155, 230–231, 297
  Liangmen point (ST 21) 94, 295
  Neiguan point (PC 6) 134, 287
  Qimen point (LV 14) 163, 291
  Rugen point (ST 18) 163, 295
  Ruzhong point (ST 17) 163, 295
  Sanyinjiao point (SP 6) 196, 293
  Shenfeng point (KI 23) 163, 296
  Shenmen point (HT 7) 129, 285
  Shuigou point (DU 26) 231, 299
  Sibai point (ST 2) 155, 230–231, 294
  Sizhukong point (SJ 23) 230–231, 288
  Taiyang point (EX-HN 5) 146, 155, 230–231, 300
  Tiantu point (RN 22) 240, 298
  Tinghui point (GB 2) 231, 292
  Wuyi point (ST 15) 163, 295
  Xiaguan point (ST 7) 231, 240, 295
  Xiongxiang point (SP 19) 163, 293
  Yanggu point (SI 5) 129–130, 286
  Yingxiang point (LI 20) 230–231, 240, 290
  Yinlingquan point (SP 9) 196, 293
  Yintang point (EX-HN 3) 230–231, 300
  Yongquan point (KI 1) 273, 296
  Yuyao point (EX-HN 4) 230–231, 300
  Zhongfu point (LU 1) 163, 289
acupuncture 14, 27, 33, 36, 54–55, 130, 135, 142, 145, 227, 247, 258, 282
acute hepatitis A 159
acute injury with muscle swelling and pain 96
aging 72–75, 86, 89, 123, 132, 147, 153, 161, 187, 200, 228, 245, 247, 249, 250–251, 263, 271
Ai Fu Tiao Jing Wan 艾附调经丸 94
allergy 68, 157, 160
almond oil (for massage) 75
almond 甜杏仁 133, 228
aloe 芦荟 76, 198
Alzheimer 260
amenorrhea 80, 92, 95, 269
American ginseng 西洋参 135
amnesia 85

anemia 82, 85, 89, 144, 171, 262
angelica dahurica 白芷 236–237
appendicitis 232
appetite (lack, low, pick, poor) 69, 82, 84–85, 87–88, 185, 199, 206
apple 苹果 123, 157
apple cider vinegar 苹果醋 170, 270, 280
artemisia capillaris 茵陈蒿 159
artichoke 蓟 165, 169, 171
asparagus 芦笋 169, 233
asparagus lettuce (celtuce) 莴笋 133
asthma 91, 100, 219–220, 227, 268
astragalus (root) 黄芪 86, 129, 135, 201–202
athlete's foot 170
avocado 鳄梨 55
azuki bean 赤小豆 105, 161, 195, 232–233

B

balding in patches 265
bamboo fungus 竹荪 162, 187
bath (foot, body) 27, 72, 76, 79, 81, 95, 126, 163, 237
beef 牛肉 161, 165, 169
beet (beetroot) 甜菜 59, 123, 171
betelnut's peel 大腹皮 204
bitter melon 苦瓜 67, 182
black tea 红茶 182, 269
blackberry 黑莓 160
bleeding 92–95, 171, 173, 179, 183, 185, 206, 226, 238, 246
blood blockage 64
blood deficiency 82, 85, 91–92, 96, 118, 126, 149–150, 152–153, 159, 169, 173, 189, 262
blood disorder 119
blood stagnation 80–81, 96, 118, 123–124, 151–152, 167, 173, 236
blood stasis 79
boat-fruited sterculia seed 胖大海 241
body hair 37, 40–41, 47–49, 211–212, 222, 224
body heat 120–121, 233
breast
- blockage 161, 163, 167
- cyst 161, 164–165
- full (distention, swelling) 50, 77, 141, 166
- late development 148
- lump (solid nodule) 163, 167
  - painful 96, 164
- mastitis 96, 166, 167
- normal development of 248
- sagging 161
- slow development 161
- sore 140
- tenderness 77, 141

breath (bad) 99, 192, 194, 206–207
broad bean 蚕豆 165
bronchitis 194, 224, 227
brown rice 糙米 187, 282
brown rice syrup 糙米浆 127, 273
brown sugar 红糖 83, 125, 128
bugbane rhizome (rhizoma cimicifugae) 升麻 202
burdock 牛蒡 198
burdock seed 牛蒡子 167
burping 70
butter 黄油 85, 164

C

capillary 60, 111, 120, 126
cancer 80, 84, 89, 93, 130, 167, 227
carrot 胡萝卜 157, 162, 164–165, 198
cassia seed 决明子 157, 203
castor oil (for massage) 263
celery 旱芹 134, 157–158
cellulite 21, 189, 192, 197–198, 203, 209
Chai tea 药草茶 269
chamomile 洋甘菊 156, 182, 234
cherry 樱桃 229
chest pressure 126
Chia 鼠尾草 198
chicken 鸡肉 70, 84, 161, 162, 164–165, 169, 174, 202, 205, 208, 248
chicory 菊苣 158
chili 辣椒 128, 280
Chinese angelica root 当归 74, 91–93, 135, 172–174
Chinese yam 山药 73, 88, 208, 272
chive seed 韭子 277
cholecystitis 159
chrysanthemum 白菊花 90, 158–160, 182, 237
cinnamon 肉桂 70, 74, 128–129, 269, 273–274, 279
citrus peel 橘皮 237
claustrophobia 264
clove 丁香 70, 74, 164, 200, 269, 276, 279
clove oil (for massage) 75
coconut oil (for massage) 75, 237
cold limb 127, 251
colitis 205
complexion
  dull 96, 153
  gloomy 153
  pale 117, 199
  radiant (glowing) 24, 26, 38, 46, 50, 109–110, 117, 127, 135, 201
  sallow 126
  yellow 153, 268
constipation 83–84, 86, 92, 100, 103, 139, 168, 198, 203–204, 220, 232, 241, 261, 267
coriander 香菜 162, 164–165
corn silk 玉米须 194, 237, 240
cou li 49
cough 48, 81–82, 84, 86, 93, 100, 204, 206, 220, 227–228, 268, 277
cracked heels 229
crystal sugar 冰糖 240
cucumber 黄瓜 74, 209
cyst 14, 161, 164–165, 236

D

dan tian area (below the belly button) 155, 255–256
dandelion 蒲公英 165–166, 233–234
dandruff 58, 75, 270
dark plum (mume fruit) 乌梅 206, 235
diabetes 89
diarrhea 69, 82, 85, 87, 90, 94, 99, 157, 173, 183, 185–186, 194, 199–200, 205–206, 232, 241, 251, 261
difficult labor 96
dizziness 64, 84, 89, 91, 104 ,117, 134, 159, 251, 267

dried bean curd 豆腐干 156
drynaria fortune 骨碎补 272
dull ache 112, 173, 251
dysentery 205, 232
dysuria 96

E

eclipta 墨旱莲 88
edema 21, 85, 96, 129–130, 181–182, 192–194, 196, 203, 251, 277
edible bird's nest 燕窝 262
egg 鸡蛋 161–163
eggplant 茄子 124
erectile dysfunction 277
erysipelas 233
eucommia bark 杜仲 90, 274
euryale seed (fox nut) 芡实 275
exhaustion 84, 168, 183, 185
eye discharge 154, 156, 158
eye
  blurred vision 39, 62, 64, 84, 98, 159–160, 168, 260
  cataract 157
  cloudy vision 154
  color blindness 62
  darkness under 133
  dryness 62, 98, 140, 159
  dull pain 154
  fatigue 63
  infection 154, 156
  itchy 140, 155–156, 157–158, 238
  myopia 62
  night blindness 157, 159
  pain 140
  pink 157
  red 98, 140, 154, 155, 157
  sensitivity to light 155
  sour 140
  sty 156
  swollen 64, 98, 158, 215
  tearful 98, 148, 155
  under bags 192, 209
  watery 155
  yellow 158–159
  yellow coloration in 155
eyebrow 21, 47, 141, 155, 230–231, 233, 237, 263, 297, 300
eyelash 47, 154, 263
eyesight (near- and far-sightedness) 89

F

face
  acne 14, 17, 50, 74, 81, 96, 105, 198, 222, 228, 234–235
  pale 26, 91–92, 112, 123, 126
  puffy 239
  red 15, 76, 119–120, 121, 126, 131, 140, 159, 234
  swelling 215
fatigue 63, 65, 82–83, 86–87, 91, 117, 123, 200, 204, 260, 268
fatty liver 132, 198
fear of heights 264
fennel 小茴香 70, 200, 269, 279
feverfew 小白菊花 182
fig 无花果 172, 197, 241, 277
Five-Element Soup 198, 206
Five Elements Theory 37, 52, 58–59, 61, 252
Five Emotions

anger 37–39, 41, 50, 134, 137–138, 140–141, 144, 152–153, 161, 168, 174–175, 302
fear 37–38, 41, 84, 101, 130, 243–244, 263–264, 302
joy 37–38, 41, 109, 302
thinking 37–38, 41, 56, 177–178, 190–191, 213, 251, 260, 302
worry 38, 211–212, 226, 263, 302
five leaf gynostemma 绞股蓝 132
five palm heat 95, 120, 159, 251
Five-White Paste 236–237
five-spice 69–70
flatstem milkvetch seed (astragali complanati) 沙苑子 277
Flos Eriocauli 谷精草 158
flu 100, 157, 280
food stagnation 152, 206
forgetful(ness) 84, 87, 98, 180, 185
fo-ti root 何首乌 73, 172, 232, 266–267
Fructus Tribuli 白蒺藜 172
fu (organ) 31–32, 34, 36, 40–42, 44, 109, 137, 177–178, 211, 220, 243, 304, 306

G

gardenia 栀子 159, 170, 172, 224
gas 70–71, 186, 200, 204
ginger 姜 69, 70, 76, 84, 88, 92, 94, 128, 157, 165, 169–170, 202, 240, 268–270, 279, 281
gingko
leaf 银杏叶 208, 239
nut 白果 134, 195, 207, 239, 275
gluey millet 秫米 133
glutinous rice 糯米 78, 88, 90, 161, 205
grape 葡萄 124, 238
green apple 青苹果 160
green tea 绿茶 73, 194, 199, 207, 214, 240
gua sha 27, 196–197, 258
gypsum (for facemask) 74, 231

H

hair
brittle 56
color change 40
dry 57, 263, 269
dull looking 56, 58
grey 15–16, 56–57, 59, 250, 263, 265, 267–268
loss 21–22, 40, 56–60, 101, 245, 249, 262–263, 265–267, 270–271
oily 58, 269
poor growth 75, 262, 266, 269, 270
seborrheic alopecia 271
split end 263
thin 56, 58, 262, 266
white 265
hawthorn berry 山楂 15, 121, 124–125, 199
hay fever 100, 155, 238–239
headache 92, 99, 104, 141
hearing (decrease, difficulty, loss, weak) 39, 86, 245, 261, 272
deafness 260
tinnitus (ringing in the ears) 39, 64,

89, 245, 251, 260–261, 267, 272
heartbeat 98, 111, 117
heartburn 83, 99
heat rash and boils 96
hemorrhoid 232, 276–277
hemp seed 火麻仁 75, 229
hemp seed oil (for massage) 229
hepatitis 233
hernia 82–83, 200, 268
hiccup 186, 200
high blood pressure 75, 89, 123, 135
high cholesterol 89, 158
honey 蜂蜜 76, 79, 88, 90, 105, 121, 162, 172, 195, 209, 229, 232, 235, 237, 266, 272, 277, 280, 282
honeysuckle 金银花 166, 234,
hot flush 120, 126, 159, 251
hysteria 84, 133

I

impotence (impotency) 83–84, 269
indigestion (or acid reflux) 32, 85, 121, 206
Indigo naturalis 青黛 233
infertility 100, 269
inflammation 47, 91, 153
irritability 82, 84, 123

J

jaundice 158, 232
jin ye (body fluid) 13, 24–27, 31, 34, 36, 40, 42, 48–49, 58–59, 62, 68, 70, 74, 86, 110–111, 118, 121, 123, 126, 138–139, 143–145, 157–160, 163, 169, 171, 179–181, 188–189, 204, 209, 214–215, 218, 222, 224–225, 228–229, 233, 239, 252, 254, 266–267, 277, 301, 306
joint (pain, weakness) 15, 92, 124, 194, 268, 273
lack of coordination 149
jujube (Chinese date) 红枣 59, 73, 82–85, 90, 127–128, 134, 161, 172, 187, 195, 205, 268

K

kalimeris indica 马兰 238
kelp 昆布 168, 181, 195
Kiwi fruit 猕猴桃 276

L

lassitude 84, 91
lavender oil (for massage) 75
leek 大蒜叶 156
lemon 柠檬 81, 105, 121, 125, 127, 168, 171, 174, 237
lentil 小扁豆 67, 199
leucopenia 233
licorice root 甘草 88, 135, 205, 232
lightheaded(ness) 38, 87, 104
lily bulb 百合 55, 86, 105, 133–134, 187, 228–229
lime 青柠 168, 170, 238
Lingzhi mushroom 灵芝 133
linseed 亚麻籽 271
lip

bleeding 206
cracked 40, 189, 206, 208–209
dry 103, 189
lusterless 40
pale 40, 189, 206–208
purple 189, 206–207
liver fire 65, 140–142
liver hyperactivity 141, 144
longan 龙眼 73, 85, 90, 161, 229, 273
loose bowel movement 84, 157
loquat 枇杷 234
lotus (leaf, plumule, seed) 荷叶 莲心 莲子 121, 195, 275
low sexual drive 276
lychee 荔枝 73, 81–83, 167–168, 199
lymph node 130

M

macadamia nut 夏威夷果 272
malt sugar 麦芽糖 127, 198
maple syrup 枫糖浆 162, 277
marine algae 海藻 181
massage 13, 18, 33, 35, 54, 60, 65, 72, 74–75, 79, 81, 128, 130, 134–135, 142, 154–155, 161, 163, 171, 174–175, 183, 196, 197, 209, 227–228, 230–231, 263, 265, 270
meditation 63, 213, 255
menstruation
dark and clotted menstrual blood 152
delay 80, 248
disturbed cycle 246
dysmenorrhea 92
early 248
heavy 81–82, 96
irregular 77, 92, 164
long 82, 94, 96
pain 80, 92, 95, 152
skipped menstrual cycles 164
too little blood flow 164
meridians
Conception Vessel (Ren) 34, 117, 202, 282–283, 298
Governing Vessel (Du) 34, 117, 282–283, 299
Jueyin Liver Meridian of Foot 35, 53, 62, 137, 145, 283, 291
Jueyin Pericardium Meridian of Hand 35, 115, 283, 287
Shaoyang Gallbladder Meridian of Foot 35, 53, 137, 145–146, 250, 283, 292
Shaoyang *San Jiao* Meridian of Hand 35, 115, 250, 288
Shaoyin Heart Meridian of Hand 35, 53, 109, 114–115, 283, 285
Shaoyin Kidney Meridian of Foot 35, 243, 256–257, 283, 296
Taiyang Bladder Meridian of Foot 35, 53, 243, 250, 256–257, 283, 297
Taiyang Small Intestine Meridian of Hand 35, 109, 114, 250, 283, 286
Taiyin Lung Meridian of Hand 35, 53, 211, 219–221, 283, 289
Taiyin Spleen Meridian of Foot 35, 177–178, 183–184, 283, 293
Yangming Large Intestine Meridian of Hand 35, 53, 211, 220–221, 249–250, 283. 290

Yangming Stomach Meridian of Foot 35, 177–178, 183–184, 249–250, 283, 294
migraine 99, 141
mint 薄荷 126, 158, 237
momordica fruit 罗汉果 241
mood swing 84, 141
motherwort 益母草 74, 95–96
plaster 益母草膏 96
powder 益母草颗粒 96
mouth
bitter taste 69, 139
canker sores 81, 208
dry 86, 120, 143, 168, 188
peeling skin and frequent cracks in the corners of 188
sticky 102, 182
sweet 102
ulcer 82, 86, 208
moxibustion 94, 282
mugwort 艾叶 74, 76, 93–94
mulberry and leaf 桑椹 桑叶 131, 158, 160, 166, 234, 267, 273
mumps 233
mung bean 绿豆 121–122, 232–234
muscle
atrophy 39, 189–190, 250
knot 99
lack of strength 190
pain 96
sagging 26, 190
shrinkage 189
sprained 170
stiffness 99
swelling 96
tears 99
tightness 99, 104
weakness 39, 91, 99, 104
mustard seed 芥子 197

N

nail
brittle 98, 150
cracked 98
fungus 170
lack shine 150
not grow 150, 169
pale 150
purple 150, 207
thin 150
vertical line 150
weak 150
nausea 75, 82, 99, 200
neck 91, 114, 145, 183, 196, 256, 283, 300
nocturnal emission 269
nose (bleed, dry, rosacea, redness, running, sinusitis, swelling) 39, 48, 224–225, 227, 237–239
numbness (legs or arms, with stiffness) 91–92, 149
nutmeg 肉豆蔻 199–200, 279

O

oat 燕麦 83, 90, 282
olive 橄榄 271
olive oil 橄榄油 158, 162, 164–165, 174, 207–209
olive vinegar 橄榄醋 158
onion 洋葱 128

Oolong tea 乌龙茶 182, 198
Tieguanyin tea 铁观音茶 198
orange oil (for massage) 197
osmanthus flower 桂花 275
osteoporosis 39, 259
oyster
sauce 蚝油 280
shell 牡蛎壳 135

P

palpitation 59, 81, 84–85, 87, 91–92, 97, 112–113, 117, 126, 229
papaya 番木瓜 86, 240
paralysis 190
parsley 西芹 157–158
parsnip 欧防风 129, 158
paste 27, 70, 72, 76, 79, 85, 88, 170, 174, 205, 229, 231, 235–237, 239, 273, 280–282
pea 豌豆 162, 164–165
peach kernel 桃仁 172–173
pear 梨 55, 229
pearl barley 薏苡仁 67, 73, 105, 194–195, 234–235
pearl powder 珍珠粉 171, 235
pei lan orchard (Herba Eupatorii) 佩兰 207
pelvic floor dysfunction 275
pepper 胡椒 164–165, 195
persimmon leaf 柿叶 174
pigmentation
after giving birth 171
birthmark 151
brown 151–152
dark 173
pregnancy 51
pimple 14, 21, 47, 49–50, 231, 234
pine nut 松子 203–204
pine nut oil 松子油 229
pneumonia 227
polyp 67, 258
pomegranate and skin 石榴 石榴皮 205–206, 276
poria 白茯苓 87–88, 237
pork 猪肉 69, 161, 165
postpartum abdominalgia 92
premature ejaculation 83
psoraleae (Psoralea corylifolia L) 补骨脂 88, 172
psoriasis 52, 233
pulse 43, 102, 112, 117, 119
pumpkin 南瓜 162
pustule 81

Q

qi
chest qi 217, 303
defensive qi 48–49, 63, 216–217, 222–224, 228, 241, 303
nutrition qi 59, 144, 217, 303
original qi 36, 49, 303
qi gong 117, 249

R

radish 萝卜 168, 198–199, 206–207
radix ampelopsis 白蔹 237
radix cynanchi auriculati (radix cynanchi wilfordi) 白首乌 236

raisin 葡萄干 276
raspberry 覆盆子 树莓 160, 268, 275
raw fo-ti root 生首乌 172
red bayberry 杨梅 205
red kidney bean 芸豆 大红豆 268
red sore 113
red wine 红酒 124, 274
Reiki 35
rhizoma bletillae 白芨 237
rhubarb root 大黄 170
rice 大米 85–86, 125, 133, 162, 187, 195, 205, 267, 276
rice vinegar 米醋 280
rice wine 米酒 161, 162, 169, 274, 280–281
root of common wild peony (radix paeoniae rubra) 赤芍 172
rose
  bud 玫瑰 73, 77–79, 126, 135, 204
  oil (for massage) 75, 79
  water 236
rosemary 迷迭香 69, 164, 269
  oil (for massage) 75
  water 269

S

sadness 37–38, 41, 54, 211–212, 226–227
safflower 红花 79–81, 172–173
  oil (for massage) 81, 197
saffron 番红花 79–81, 173
seaweed 紫菜 168, 181
seminal emission 246, 264, 269, 275, 277
sesame 芝麻 16, 78, 266–267, 273
  oil 麻油 164–165, 207, 280
schisandra berry (Chinese magnolivine fruit) 五味子 272
shen 110, 112–113
shiitake mushroom 香菇 159–160, 198
shortness of breath 84, 86, 92, 100, 104, 203, 268
Sichuan pepper 四川花椒 194–195, 279
silver ear (tremella, white fungus) 银耳 55, 73, 76, 85–86, 121, 123, 228–229, 240
sinus 20, 100, 224, 228, 237, 239, 272
skin
  blemish 20, 175, 211, 228
  burns 232
  carbuncle 96, 232
  couperose 126
  dull 26, 112, 229
  eczema 47, 52, 233
  irritated 23
  itchiness 49, 95, 232
  oily 103, 105, 182, 223, 234, 240
  raised lump 228
  rash 14–15, 49, 222, 232
  rough 43, 48, 93, 96, 133, 239
  saggy 26, 51, 192, 200
  scald 232
  sensitive 75, 228, 232–233, 236
  spider vein 49, 54, 120, 123–124, 235
  warts 228, 235
  wrinkle 22, 51, 82, 105, 117, 133, 153, 155, 197, 223, 228–229, 235, 249–250
  yellow tinge 23, 139

skin zones 52–54
sleep
disorder 60
disturbance 98, 114, 127, 133
inability to 119, 130
insomnia 59, 84–85, 87, 89, 91–92, 113–114, 126, 133
light 84
nightmare 89, 98
poor quality of 59, 134
with the eyes half open 63
solid nodule 161, 167–168
soy sauce 酱油 169, 280
spinach 菠菜 59, 171
Spiritual Axis (*Ling Shu Jing*) 60
sprained tendon 170
spring onion 葱 169, 207, 238, 273, 279, 281
star anise 八角 70, 273
starch 淀粉 88, 204
stemona tuberosa lour 百部 170
stomach
cold 69, 83, 85, 121, 142, 157, 186, 199
distention 83–84
fullness 32, 103
stomach ache (pain) 78, 82, 85, 199
stool
dry 103, 203, 267
incomplete evacuation 182
loose 69, 93, 103, 173
soft 87
watery 157
weak, difficult excretion 92
sugar intolerance 71
sweating
continuous 222–223
emotional or nervous 40
excess 48, 135
night 95
spontaneous 39, 48, 222–223
sword bean 刀豆 268

T

tai ji 249, 262
tangerine leaf 橘叶 165
tangerine skin 陈皮 88, 204
taro 芋头 164–165
TCM body clock 44, 304
thirst 81–82, 84, 86, 90, 95, 101, 113, 120, 123, 140, 141, 143, 157, 168, 229, 233, 277
throat 82, 90, 100, 103, 120, 166, 183, 214, 217, 220, 224, 226, 228, 239, 241, 256, 277
thrombus 91
tincture 27, 72, 88, 201
tiredness 84
tongue
pale (with white fur) 92, 102, 112, 118, 126, 193
purple 104, 112, 152
purple dots 104, 112, 173
red spots (or sores) 118
red with no coating 120
red with yellow coating 120, 126
redness on the tip 113
toothache 82
tui na 130, 258
tumour 207
turmeric 姜黄 272

U

ulcer 82, 86, 92, 98, 113, 118, 123, 131, 208
urinary incontinence 269
urine
chronic infections 275
frequent 88, 253
involuntary 264
scanty 87, 103, 120
yellow 120, 159, 168, 257
uterine bleeding 92

V

vaginal blood discharge after child delivery 96
vertigo 91, 229
vinegar 醋 88, 158, 186, 208, 237, 270, 280
vitamin E capsule 75, 76
vitiligo 51, 172
voice (hoarse, weak) 39, 226, 241, 277
vomiting 194, 199

W

walnut 核桃 16, 203, 266–269, 276
watermelon 西瓜 74, 121, 131, 208, 235, 254
weight
overweight 197–198, 203
underweight 68, 199
weight loss 120, 235
well salt 井盐 181
wheat flour 面粉 170
white spot 152, 170, 172
willow branch 柳枝 271
wind heat 154–158
winter melon 冬瓜 193–195, 215, 238–239
wolfberry (goji berry) 枸杞子 55, 59, 74, 88–90, 105, 160, 172, 187, 209, 229, 268, 271
wood ear (black fungus) 黑木耳 59, 208, 235, 268, 277

Y

yang deficiency 69, 93, 118, 128, 167, 197, 199, 201, 203, 265, 266
yang weakness 199, 251
Yang Yuhuan 20
Yellow Emperor's Canon (*Huang Di Nei Jing*) 62, 64, 138, 146, 212, 246, 247
yin deficiency 93, 95, 118, 157, 159, 167, 174, 238, 251, 252, 266
yin weakness 82, 120, 143, 199
ylang ylang 依兰 75
yogurt 酸奶 76

Z

zang (organ) 31, 32, 34, 40, 41, 42, 44, 109, 137, 171, 177, 178, 211, 220, 243, 302, 306
Zhao Feiyan 20

Standard Meridian Abbreviations
HT: Heart Meridian (heart system) SI: Small Intestine Meridian (heart system) PC: Pericardium Meridian (heart system) SJ: *San Jiao* Meridian (heart system)
LV: Liver Meridian (liver system) GB: Gallbladder Meridian (liver system)
SP: Spleen Meridian (spleen system) ST: Stomach Meridian (spleen system)
LU: Lung Meridian (lung system) LI: Large Intestine Meridian (lung system)
KI: Kidney Meridian (kidney system) BL: Bladder Meridian (kidney system)

Cold Constitution

Symptoms

Sensitive to cold; cold limbs; prefers ᴡarm drinks; little or no sweating; pale or ıffy complexion; drinks too much cold ter or green tea; eats too many vegetables ruits

Recommendations

amon stick (BL, HT, LU), ginger (LU, SP, ST), uan pepper (SP, ST, KI), fennel (LV, KI, SP, ST), sword bean (ST, KI), rose bud (LV, SP), kumquat (LV, SP, ST), clove (SP, ST, LU, KI), mustard (ST, LU), leek (LV); mugwort leaf (LV, SP, KI)

ds
ryone

.I), almond e (HT, LU, SP, .U,SP), gingko nflower seeds (SP, KI, HT), (LU, ST, KI), P, LU, LI, LV), T), beet root shiitake ms (LV,)

irst; e

Damp Constitution

Symptoms

Oily hair or skin; prone to skin pimples; loose stool or turbid urine; heaviness in the muscles or head; sleepy; large quantity of excretion (eyes, nose ears); edema; frequently drinks or smokes; sticky taste in mouth; dislikes sugar with tea or dairy

Food Recommendations

Pearl barley (SP, ST, LU), green tea (HT, LU, KI, ST), pumpkin (SP, ST, LU), grapes (LU, SP, KI), marine algae (LV, ST, KI), button mushrooms (LU, HT, SP), celery (LV, ST, LU), kumquat (LV, SP, ST), garlic (SP, ST, LU, LI), papaya (LU, ST), chicory (LV), asparagus lettuce (LI, ST), poria (HT, SP, LU, KI)

Weak Constitution

Symptoms

Easily tired; low voice or a dislike of talking; muscles are soft and weak; prone to numbness or sagging skin; lightheaded; irregular or interrupted elimination; frequent shortness of breath; prone to sinus problems

Food Recommendations

Astragalus (SP, LU), Chinese yam (LU, SP, KI), cherry (SP, KI), jujube (SP, ST, HT), spinach (LV, ST, SI, LI), longan (HT, SP), lychee (LV, SP), American ginseng (LU, HT, KI, SP), wolfberry (LV, KI, LU), walnut (KI, LU, LI), raspberry (LV, KI), cinnamon bark (KI, SP, HT, LV), dry ginger (LU, SP, ST, KI, HT), mulberry fruit (LV, KI), chive seed (KI, LV), angelica (LV, HT, SP)

A Useful Guide to Foods and Herbs: Considering Constitution and Organ System

Over its long history, Chinese medicine has come to realize that different foods enter specific meridian pathways, directing their effect towards particular organs. When we know which meridian and/or organ a food will target, this is useful in treating a disorder of that particular organ system. Another approach to choosing food is to do so according to the body constitution. To maximize the benefits, use these ingredients for at least one month.

Heat Constitution

Symptoms

Sensitive to heat; prefers cold drinks; sweats a lot; irritable; flushed complexion or rash; drinks too much coffee; eats too much red meat and spicy food

Food Recommendations

Mint (LU, LV), mung bean (HT, LV, ST), watermelon (HT, ST, BL), chrysanthemum (LU, LV), cassia seed (LV, LI), honeysuckle (LU, HT, ST), dandelion (LV, ST), aloe (LV, ST, LI), loquat (LU, SP), kelp (KI, LV), dolichols seed (SP, ST), asparagus (LV), lotus plumule (HT, KI), celery (LV, ST, LU), gardenia (HT, LV, LU, ST, SJ), eggplant (SP, ST, LI)

Overly Strong Constitution

Symptoms

Not easy to relax; consumes high quantities of meat; muscles are tight and sore; fullness in the head; pressure or distention in the chest; infrequent elimination; frequently excited; dark or purple lips or tongue bodyd thick tongue fur

Food Recommendations

Peach fruit (LU, LI), peach kernel (LV, HT, LI), safflower (HT, LV), vinegar (LV, ST), turnip (ST), hawthorn (SP, ST, LV), tangerine (SP, LU, ST, LV, GB), azuki bean (HT, SI, SP), chive leaf (KI, LU, ST, LV), turmeric (SP, LV), mulberry leaf (LU, LV), motherwort (LV, KI, PC)

Dry Constitution

Symptoms

Dry or cracked skin; dry, thin, and dull hair; dry stool; constipation or scanty urine; dryness in the sense organs; t anxiety; prone to skin wrinkles; thin body fig

Food Recommendations

Honey (LU, SP, LI), lily bulb (LU, HT), sesam (LV, KI, SP, LI), apple (HT, LU, ST), oyster (L HT), flaxseed (LU, LV, LI), lemon (ST, LU), peas (SP, ST), persimmon (HT, LU, LI), soybean (SP, ST, LI), potato (KI, SP, ST), millet (LU, ST, LI)

Fo for Ev

Fig (LU, ST, (LU, LI), licori ST), carrot (LV, nut (LU, KI), s (LU, LI), lotu white fungu black fungus (olives (LU, (HT, LV) mushrc S

F w or

Foo

Cin Sic